Managerialism and Nursing

Over the past decade, government reform of the health service has dramatically increased managerial control over the traditional professions of medicine and nursing. In the wake of these reforms, *Managerialism and Nursing* looks at the effect of new management activity on nurses, and documents the struggle to define the core values of health care.

Based on an innovative study of nurses and their managers, the book examines the relationship between the two by looking at the contrasting ways in which each group argues its case and presents its identity. While many of nursing's leaders have promoted nursing as a rational and cost-effective activity, nurses given voice in this book express strongly held notions of duty and self-sacrifice. Michael Traynor gives a fluent account of postmodern theories and aptly demonstrates their value in understanding the struggle to present a unified voice and be heard that is inherent in nursing's history.

Managerialism and Nursing makes a significant contribution to debates about nursing and its claims to power and influence. It provides stimulating reading for anyone interested in the future of the health service and also serves as a highly readable introduction to postmodern approaches to analysis.

Michael Traynor studied English Literature before qualifying as a nurse and a health visitor. He is a lecturer at the Centre for Policy in Nursing Research at the London School of Hygiene and Tropical Medicine.

Managerialism and Nursing

Beyond oppression and profession

Michael Traynor

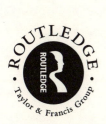

London and New York

First published 1999 by Routledge
11 New Fetter Lane, London EC4P 4EE

Simultaneously published in the USA and Canada
by Routledge
29 West 35th Street, New York, NY 10001

Routledge is an imprint of the Taylor & Francis Group

© 1999 Michael Traynor

Typeset in Galliard by Keystroke, Jacaranda Lodge, Wolverhampton
Printed and bound in Great Britain by St Edmundsbury Press,
Bury St Edmunds, Suffolk.

British Library Cataloguing in Publication Data
A catalogue record for this book is available from the British Library

Library of Congress Cataloguing in Publication Data
Traynor, Michael, 1956–
    Managerialism and nursing : beyond oppression and profession /
Michael Traynor.
        p.   cm.
    Includes bibliographical references and index.
    1. Nurses—Supervision of—Great Britain. 2. Nursing services—
Great Britain—Administration. 3. Interprofessional relations—
Great Britain. 4. Nurse administrators—Great Britain.
5. Conflict management—Great Britain. 6. Nursing services—Great
Britain—Personnel management. I. Title.
    [DNLM: 1. Nursing—organization & administration—Great Britain.
2. Interprofessional Relations. 3. Nurse Administrators. WY 105
T783m 1999]
RT86.45.T73 1999
362.1′73′068—dc21
DNLM/DLC
                                                    98–42097
                                                    CIP

ISBN 0–415–17895–9 (hbk)
ISBN 0–415–17896–7 (pbk)

To my two small friends,
Dante and Gamaliel
and to the memory of my father,
George Hugh Traynor

Contents

Tables

Preface

In 1991 the United Kingdom (UK) government introduced reforms of the National Health Service (NHS), part of a series of rationalisations aimed at increasing accountability and responsiveness, and containing the service's costs. These rationalisations featured the strengthening of managerial control over the traditional professions, among them medicine and nursing, a system of contracting between purchasers and providers of health care and unprecedented attention to the control and measurement of inputs, particularly in terms of employees' activities.

This book grew out of concerns arising from my involvement in a study of nursing morale and managerial strategy in the wake of these reforms. The study took place in four first wave NHS Trusts working in the community sector and ran over four years.

The discovery that nurses and managers described themselves in strong, and sometimes hostile, opposition to each other led me to develop this as a framework for analysis of the whole situation. Influenced by postmodern philosophy, deconstructive literary theory and discourse analysis, I began to investigate the way that each group argued its case and presented its identity.

Postmodern writers argue that reason and rationality have come to be defined in terms that support the values and interests of particular groups and marginalise other groups, undermining their claims to knowledge. In this study managers tended to characterise, at least sections of, their nursing workforce as irrational, fearful and traditional. Nurses described themselves in terms of moral agency and self-sacrifice in the face of exploitation by their managers.

This critique, effected through literary approaches, is offered as a theoretical framework within which to understand, not just struggles in health services, but wider changes in Western society.

Acknowledgements

I would like to thank the Royal College of Nursing, where I was employed as a research officer in the Daphne Heald Research Unit during the fieldwork from which this project sprang, and Dr Barbara Wade, the director of the Research Unit, for tolerating my persistent inability to return from fieldwork with 'the facts'.

I am indebted to Professor Jane Robinson, my PhD supervisor, for granting that absolutely vital permission for me to take flight with my project, for providing continued critical response to the emerging work, encouragement and confidence and for first mentioning, casually, the word 'deconstruction'. I also thank all the staff in the Department of Nursing and Midwifery Studies at Nottingham for their feedback and support, and Professor Judith Parker from the University of Melbourne for encouraging me to remain a free-floating troublemaker.

I must also express my gratitude to the NHS Trust managers who gave their time and were prepared to participate in this research and risk total mis-representation at a time of political sensitivity and to the many community nurses who contributed their often painful comments and insights to this research.

Many individuals have dropped important ideas in my path during this project and well before it. Steve Shaw of College House had a key role in setting me out on a journey from religious dogmatism to philosophical thought. He also shouted down the name Richard Rorty from the roof of my house while nailing down new slates. Joanna Latimer introduced me to the work of Bruno Latour and some of the insights revealed by ethnomethodology; her own rigorous work has continually challenged me. Anne Marie Rafferty is the director of the Centre for Policy in Nursing Research where I work and I am particularly thankful for her limitless intellectual curiosity and her encouragement. She also commented on a draft of the first chapter.

Other individuals have spared their time to discuss this project, among them Ray Jobling (remarkably accessible) and Christopher Norris (20 minutes in a smoke-filled room in Cardiff on the hottest day in 1995). Also painters Hephzibah Rendle-Short and Andrew Vass have discussed notions of representa-tion and equivalence which are equally relevant to their work and to this enquiry.

I chose an expert paediatric cardiologist, Kate Bull, for advice about inserting my ideas into the reader's heart in the book's last pages. Hephzibah Rendle-Short also commented on a draft of parts of the final chapter.

The quotations from Leonard Cohen's novel *Beautiful Losers* appear by kind, and I suspect, puzzled, permission of Stranger Management Inc. and Black Spring Press. I fantasised getting a late night transatlantic call from the gravelly grocer of despair – but it never happened.

1 Introduction:
Enlightenment, rationality
and colonisation

In a passage from a troubling novel, Leonard Cohen describes the French Jesuits' attempts to convert the animist North American Iroquois to Christianity. The canny Indians cover their ears so as not to hear the discourse of sin and judgement. The Jesuits, however, take recourse to drawing lurid pictures of the torments of hell, the inhabitants of which are recognisable Iroquois.

'Take your fingers out of your ears,' said le P. Jean Pierron, first permanent missionary at Kahnawaké. 'You won't be able to hear me if you keep your fingers in your ears.'

'Ha, ha,' chuckled the ancient members of the village, who were too old to learn new tricks. 'You can lead us to water but you can't make us drink, us old dogs and horses.'

'Remove those fingers immediately!'

The priest went back to his cabin and took out his paints, for he was a skilled artist. A few days later he emerged with his picture, a bright mandala of the torments of hell. All the damned had been portrayed as Mohawk Indians. . . .

'Now, my children, this is what awaits you. Oh, you can keep your fingers where they are. . . . '

'Arghhh!'

The colours of the picture were red, white, black, orange, green, yellow and blue. . . .

'Arghhh!'

'That's right, pull them right out,' the priest invited them. 'And don't put them back. You must never put them back again. . . . '

As those waxy digits were withdrawn a wall of silence was thrown up between the forest and the hearth, and the old people gathered at the priest's hem shivered with a new kind of loneliness. They could not hear the raspberries breaking into domes, they could not smell the numberless pine needles combing out the wind, they could not remember the last moment of a trout as it lived between a flat white pebble on the streaked bed of a stream and the fast shadow of a bear claw. Like children who listen in vain to the sea in plastic sea shells they sat bewildered.

(Cohen 1993: 81–82)

Cohen pictures, with the novel's characteristic comic strip dialogue, the colonisation of the Iroquois as the moment when they allow themselves to hear the voices of the French. In that instant, echoing the fall of Adam and Eve in the Garden of Eden, they become isolated from the various magics of nature, lost to their ancient identity, bewildered.

This is a story of a similar colonisation, although the struggle is not over, and since post-structuralism, any notions of oppressor and oppressed as fixed and exclusive categories have become problematised. There may be less brutality in the story that I will develop, but there is pain and confusion alongside the evangelising activities of those who bring a new vision to sweep away fear and superstition. This is a story of an ascending rationality in UK health care and a response to it by a number of nurses. It is a rationality which I will argue finds its distant but vivid origins in the Enlightenment discovery of reason that took hold of European thought, imagination and aspiration in the eighteenth century. However, this account does not idealise any primitive state or alternative view. There is no championing of an oppressed group. What it does is make visible the contingencies behind a dominant rationality; it critiques the loss of space for difference in the wake of this powerful vision. Documenting the local exercise of power, the story places the discourses that have caught up health service managers into the contexts of economic rationalism and the modernism of Enlightenment thought. Countermovements in the story are to be found in the discourses taken up by nurses involved in care delivery and middle management. Their discourses are, in a sense, out of tune with both the rationality of management and the aspirations to power of their own professional leaders, many of whom have committed themselves to 'speaking the manager's language' perhaps to preserve their own professional, and personal, position and influence.

When I say colonisation, I intend to ask how far managerialist language and the categories of thought that this has made available, and those that it has effaced, have succeeded in establishing themselves as the dominant language of nursing within the health care professions. Effectiveness, cost-effectiveness, division of labour, the measurement of outcome, productivity, customer satisfaction, rational(ised) evidence-based practice are all now 'natural' features of nursing discourse. Nursing may offer different conclusions to managers, for example over workforce profiling, but how far it has been successfully enrolled by these criteria is a matter for argument. The words of nurses quoted in this book may represent a rapidly marginalised or even by now virtually extinct position.

This story is also a deliberate subversion of other stories. It is an exploration of deconstruction's discovery that a single text can be used to support seemingly irreconcilable positions. A deliberate subversion of the initial or face reading of a text informs the treatment of interviews and other utterances produced within this research. This involves an analysis of metaphor and its place in argument, an interrogation of a text's dualisms and a radical approach to the question of intention and context. It is also a subversion of a research approach which is based upon a number of Enlightenment premises. The most influential has been the belief in the transparency of the individual who stands in a direct relationship to the objects that he or she observes. The aims of the original research project from which this work grew were the measurement of the morale of community nurses and the gathering of information from their managers. It was based on notions of the possibility of the objectivity of measurement and the transparency of language. Its intention was to trace lines of cause and effect between government policy, managerial activity and the morale of the nursing workforce and to enable the two groups, workers and management, to understand each other better and in that sense contribute to organisational and social progress. These beliefs and intentions are problematised in this work.

Why such deliberate awkwardness, such refusal to offer constructive help at a time when it is so badly needed? And why such reluctance to champion the cause of an oppressed group such as nurses? The answers, albeit uneasy ones, stem from an ambivalence toward an Enlightenment faith in processes of emancipation and, perhaps more importantly, from a belief in the inescapability of the projects of power. First, it is the tyranny implicit in the 1980s and 1990s managerialist project that is critiqued here (and already I cannot help but refer to humanistic notions of injustice and human dignity brought into focus by the Enlightenment), not the more-or-less usefulness of rational thought as a tool with which humans can meet some of their needs. It is the denial, the marginalising, the calling into service of other types of knowledge and being that is critiqued. Second, to bring out into the open delegitimised knowledges runs the risk of their recolonisation by an ascendant discourse. I view with unease the (albeit slim) possibility that this book might make nurses easier to manage for reasons quite apart from a regard for professional autonomy. After all, Barthes urges us to not fear annexation of our words by power and its culture but neither to be naive about this possibility (Barthes 1996). Third, and on the issue of motivation, this book is not, for the most part, a calling into question of the motivation or conscious intention of either managers or health workers, nor an attempt to discredit them. Nor will it be argued that they are 'dupes', passive before the structural forces of language and thought. It is rather an examination of how certain discourses give rise to subject positions that we might find each group standing within. Finally, if this work fails to take up the cause of nurses as an occupational group, it is through a reluctance to be colonised by yet another professionalising discourse. It is easy to speak of nurses as an oppressed group for any one of a number of reasons including those of economics, gender and culture. Professionalising forces within nursing have repeatedly called upon these discourses as well as upon discourses of empowerment and epistemology in their bids for political and professional power/survival. There is a problematic relationship between, for example, moves to increase the status of nursing as one particular occupational group (vis-à-vis other occupational groups) and those which might affect the status of all women.

Nurses have responded in a mixed way to analyses of power that insist on its ubiquity, such as those offered by Foucault (1980a). I will argue in Chapter 4 that many nurses and their leaders are more inclined to present themselves as seeking liberation from oppression than they are to understand themselves as implicated in maintaining the associations between profession and power. We could understand talk of holism, patient advocacy, professionalism or feminism as notions brought in, not necessarily consciously, to support such a project. Nevertheless, such attempts have only ever been partially successful. Nursing seems to have always struggled even for control over preparation for practice. For example, in early 1999 Health Secretary Frank Dobson dropped heavy hints that the profession's elitist educational aspirations were at least partly to blame for a national nursing shortage and that nursing education may be moved, against the will of most nurses – certainly its leaders – out of the university sector back to hospitals.

Nevertheless, if this work has little to offer the professionaliser, I hope that it may be of use to some of those individuals who were involved in this research, and others like them, who found the changes affecting their work during the early and mid-1990s deeply troubling but who did not have the vocabulary to articulate their feelings. They felt, perhaps, that it would have been churlish to criticise a managerial project which was so well defined and rational and which had such good intentions. Some nurses in 'middle-management' positions come first to mind. It is for these individuals and groups, who are becoming increasingly marginalised within nursing itself, that an account is offered of how a particular discourse has become dominant and of some of the limitations of that discourse.

Horkheimer argued that the purpose of critical theory 'is not, either in its conscious intention or in its objective significance, the better functioning of any element in the structure [of capitalist society]' (Horkheimer 1972: 207). It is, rather, a concern with the way that present social arrangements fail to meet, what he terms, human needs (ibid.).

In this chapter I will introduce:

- three of the basic notions which this book employs: Enlightenment, rationality and colonisation;
- the policy context of the study and its effects on nursing;
- the approach and aims of the research from which this work grew.

ENLIGHTENMENT

'What is Enlightenment?' asks Foucault (1984b), echoing and exploring Kant's question posed two hundred years earlier in the German periodical, *Berlinische Monatschrift*. He suggests Kant argued that:

> Enlightenment is a process that releases us from the status of 'immaturity.' And by 'immaturity,' he means a certain state of our will that makes us accept someone else's authority to lead us in areas where the use of reason is called for.
>
> (ibid.: 34)

Foucault maintained that Kant viewed the Enlightenment both as a phenomenon, an ongoing historical process, and as a task and an obligation faced by all humanity. It was seen as a new stage in the evolution of humankind, and enabled people to claim a new confidence, a new authority through the operation of reason and its principles. Enlightenment is thus both a teleological project, one that concerns itself with questions about the overarching development and purpose of human existence, and the quintessential emancipatory project, hence the difficulty experienced by anyone who wishes to reject the globalising pretensions of reason but preserve the desire for emancipation. Enlightenment promised emancipation from the primitive forces of unreason in its various forms, superstition, as well as unreasonable law and religion. Kant was obliged to present his views to Frederick II in a particularly careful form, suggesting that the obedience of subjects would be ensured if the 'political principle that must be obeyed itself be in conformity with universal reason' (Foucault 1984b: 37).

The Enlightenment is also a project asserting the autonomy of the human subject rather than a relationship of dependence upon God or to abstract metaphysical principles. It is a project that still consumes a vast amount of energy and its heritage offers perhaps one reason for the persuasiveness of the 'New Right' vision of the freedom of the individual (Hayek 1967; Nozick 1974). Autonomy is also central to the claims of the modern professional and to the aspirations of the leader of the modern organisation. It is a notion mentioned a great many times by managers in this study and competing bids for this precious attribute provided a rich source of tension between them and other professionals.

RATIONALITY

The term 'rationality' as used in this book is related to the Enlightenment's reason in a number of ways. First, I have considered managers to be invoking it when they have contrasted some, fearful, authority-following, self-interested or primitive way of being with a particular mode of (non)decision-making, understanding or motivation. Second, reason claims a certain freedom from context, a certain objectivity or universal applicability. Practical reason, according to Kant, 'employs no criterion external to itself. It appeals to no content derived from experience . . . It is the essence of reason that it lays down principles which both can and ought to be held by all people, independent of circumstances and conditions' (MacIntyre 1985: 45). Kant based his moral philosophy on the principle that if the rules of morality were rational, they must be the same for all rational beings as are, for example, the rules of arithmetic. So reason is characterised by certain universalising claims, in this book, on the part of managers or nurses. Third, because such universalising claims are potentially tyrannical, its activity is noted whenever claims to a particular rationality or objectivity form the basis of the exercise of power by one group over another. Perhaps the present study could be located within the field of interest of:

a line of thinkers stretching from Max Weber to Martin Heidegger through Theodor Adorno and Max Horkheimer. Each of these men, in different ways recognised both a centrality and a danger in the process of increasing rationalisation and technological development in the world. Each also differentiated between types of reason or thinking – instrumental, substantive, formal, critical etc. – and attempted to separate out those dimensions and consequences of rational activity which were pernicious and those which in some form or other could serve as instruments of resisting or overcoming the destructive functioning of reason in Western culture.

(Rabinow 1984: 13)

In this book I have tried to deal with rationality in four ways. First, with postmodernist writer Jean François Lyotard, this book 'wages war' (Lyotard 1979: 82) against the totalising aspect of some of the particular forms of rationality found in modern health care. Second, I contrast a certain 'utilitarian' rationality of the kind propounded by Jeremy Bentham (see Chapter 2, p. 38) with the more 'deontological' (Seedhouse 1993) values of the nurses involved in this study, although there are hazards in making such a clear distinction. The nurses, I will argue, can be understood as among the sort of groups which Richard Rorty has suggested have been excluded from an objectivity or rationality that has been conceived of in terms of 'general agreement among sane and rational men' (Rorty 1980: 337). Third, with Foucault, this book undertakes an 'ascending' analysis of the local effects of rationality – power and knowledge – of 'how things work at the level of on-going subjugation' (Foucault 1980b). Fourth, in line with a literary deconstructive tendency, it analyses its material in the light of the argument that a text can be used to support apparently irreconcilable positions (Miller 1976).

COLONISATION

The third theme upon which this book draws is that of colonisation. Given the totalising ambitions of the rationality described above, this is unsurprising. Colonisation has been an image used by, for example, feminists to express the situation of being seen as an 'Other', an object for study, definition and redefinition by a dominant and dominating force (Hartsock 1990). An early example of this kind of theorising is Simone de Beauvoir's observation that men understand and describe themselves as the norm or the 'One' from which they constitute woman as the 'Other', who is defined in relation to her deviation from the male norm (De Beauvoir 1953). Many in nursing have taken up these arguments for the compelling reason that nursing's place in health care as a marginalised Other with regard to 'mainstream' medicine, acts as a vivid embodiment of societal relations between women and men. If women at large are the irrational, instinctual and dependent foil for men's rationality of detachment, then nurses fulfil the same purpose by allowing medicine's self-definition as scientific and autonomous all the more power. 'No identity can ever exist by itself and without an array of opposites, negatives, oppositions: Greeks always require barbarians' (Said 1993: 60). Links can be formed between European voyages of discovery and settlement characteristic of the eighteenth and nineteenth centuries and that other European project of thought alluded to above. Edward Said argues that 'European culture gained in strength and identity by setting itself off against the Orient as a sort of surrogate and even underground self' (Said 1978: 3). The coloniser is at once the Western historically located imperialist 'implanting . . . settlements on distant territory' (Said 1993: 8) and the supposedly transcendental Enlightenment subject surveying the world. 'Others', according to Nancy Hartsock, 'are not seen as fellow individual members of the human community, but rather as part of a chaotic, disorganised, and anonymous collectivity' (Hartsock 1990: 161) They are everything the coloniser is not. The power of the coloniser's theorising (accentuated by the promise of force) is so authoritative that they even create the 'structure of feeling' for the colonised (Said 1993: 14).

Writing about the imperialist frame of reference of Joseph Conrad's novel *Heart Of Darkness*, and about the European, Kurtz, in the African continent, Said argues that 'The circularity, the perfect closure of the whole thing is not only aesthetically but also mentally unassailable' (Said 1993: 26). The present book is an attempt to interrupt this circularity and examine the mechanisms of colonisation that use and in turn are used by discourses of rationality and independence that originate in the Enlightenment. On one level, those with political and organisational power colonise those with less by creating a frame of reference so pervasive that they are drawn to evaluate their activity and their thoughts by its criteria. The colonised take up the language and categories of the coloniser in order to present and understand themselves in ways that will be recognised and valued. I will argue that in the organisations under study, nurses involved in this research appeared largely to resist this colonisation while their managers and perhaps their professional leaders have allowed themselves to be drawn onto the ground of the coloniser. On another level, then, these discourses colonise all who locate themselves within them. On yet another level, my own explanations, legitimised by the context in which they are located, can be seen as a manifestation of the perhaps unavoidable power imbalance inherent in the process of research.

Perhaps the 1980s' and 1990s' turn to a discourse of market forces within Western public sector organisations can be understood as a turning inwards of the last century's mercantile ethos with its sense of 'all but unlimited opportunities for commercial advancement abroad' (Said 1993: 14), a colonisation of more and more fields of human activity.

Enrolment and translation are related to the notion of colonisation (Callon *et al.* 1986). For Callon and colleagues, who have studied science and technology, a particular actor (perhaps a company) 'enrols' others by defining and distributing roles, by displacing others so that they are forced to follow an itinerary that has been imposed on them, and are drawn into the logic and project of a particular 'actor-world'. For these writers an inanimate technology such as a battery cell is as likely to be enrolled in a particular project as an individual or a national corporation.

Turning from these broader themes, I will now examine the immediate policy and political background to the events which gave rise to this study.

A POLICY CONTEXT AND BUREAUCRATIC DISCOURSE

From the end of the 1970s to the mid- to late 1990s politics have been characterised by the rise of 'New Right' governments and ideologies on an almost global scale. We have seen the long incumbency of the Conservatives (under Margaret Thatcher and John Major) in the UK and the Republicans (under Ronald Reagan and George Bush) in the US, and the 'fall' of communism in Eastern Europe. Socialist beliefs have been widely understood to have become less credible (Norris 1990b) while 'individual freedom' and 'the minimal state' have continually been talked up and, to a lesser extent, perhaps, brought into being. A central feature of 'New Right' thinking was its adoption by both politicians (Brown and Sparks 1989) and theorists (Hayek 1967) of eighteenth- and nineteenth-century classical political economists' arguments against state intervention. The notion of the minimal state assumes that all that is not under state control is the proper realm of 'the market', where economically active individuals can freely pursue their own interests and profit. The paradox within such a situation is that if organisations like the NHS are taken within the machinery of the state, then the state must accept responsibility for their activities and failings. It is exactly this culpability that Conservative governments during the late 1980s and 1990s sought to avoid.

With a relatively new Labour government (since 1997) in the UK, it is too early to say whether a new *weltanshaung* will develop. The contributors to a 1997 issue of *Health Care Analysis* devoted to socialist health care reached consensus on the fact that 'whatever comes next [in UK and US health care] is very unlikely to be socialist – there are just too many theoretical and practical difficulties in the way' (Seedhouse 1997). The deep shift that we have witnessed since the end of the 1970s in Western consciousness goes beyond the political colour of the dominating party. Nevertheless, documents such as the 1997 White Paper (Department of Health 1997) feature a conscious replacement of the language and structures of competition with more co-operative talk.

In the UK the financial turmoil created in the wake of the 1976 oil crisis and what has been described as the failure of the welfare state to fulfil its more optimistic expectations created an unavoidable context for policy that followed (Brown and Sparks 1989). Within this context, UK health policy can be understood as the bringing in of successive waves of rationality with the aim, on the part of government, of controlling large numbers of NHS employees who were acting as if they were autonomous individuals (Pollitt 1993). At the forefront of these groups were doctors whose activities had ever growing implications for expenditure.

Rising public spending, which was already receiving attention under a previous Labour administration, came in for particular scrutiny under the incoming Conservative regime in 1979 (Pollitt 1991). In addition, one policy commentator argues that many conservatives saw in the very principles of the NHS 'many of the manifestations of Britain's supposed post-war malaise: the heavy influence of central and local bureaucracies, the restrictive practices of powerful professions, the absence of real consumer choice; the lack of incentives for innovation and efficiency; and the deadening reliance upon government funds' (Butler 1992: 1). To make matters worse, 'a public service bureaucracy dominated by a profession or set of professions was a double evil – a budget-maximising monopolist that was likely to be both unnecessarily costly and deeply inadequate' (Pollitt 1993: 43). Solutions to these problems were sought from within the practices of private sector organisations with their presumed efficiency. The discourses of 'managerialism' and of market-type competition began to make their way into the public sector from industry and commerce. In the UK NHS, a series of 'scrutinies' by Sir Derek Rayner, from the retail chain Marks & Spencer, were introduced in 1982 (ibid.) and the following year another figurehead from the commercial world, Sir Roy Griffiths, from the Sainsbury supermarket chain, was called upon to chair an inquiry into NHS management (Strong and Robinson 1990).

Calling the autonomous to account

Griffiths' central claim was that the NHS lacked clear chains of control and accountability. The light that he was going to shed on this gloomy state of affairs was to recommend the introduction of general management. He proposed general managers at regional, district and unit level employed on short-term contracts. Subsequently these managers were faced with the extra incentives of performance-related pay and individual performance review. Such arrangements 'link[ed] the personal objectives of individual managers with corporate – and ultimately ministerial – objectives for the service as a whole' (Wistow 1992: 106). However, no drive for greater efficiency and control would be complete without some measure to limit the clinical freedom of doctors within the service – a freedom which had formed one of the foundational agreements at the very instigation of the NHS. Griffiths sought to closely involve doctors in management, to persuade them to 'accept the management responsibility which goes with clinical freedom' (Griffiths 1983: para. 8.2) – and who can be seen to shun responsibility? Schemes like the resource management initiative (RMI) had this as their aim.

In spite of such measures, some argued that the impact of the changes was limited, that 'management stop[ped] at the consulting room door' (Harrison *et al.* 1989). However, more recently, some commentators have seen the incorporation of professionals into management roles as an effective method of controlling, and colonising, professional activity and consciousness:

In the 'old days' the NHS hospital could sometimes seem to exist *for* the doctors, rather than the other way round. Pre-Griffiths administrators saw their role as one of *facilitating* the work of doctors and nurses, not controlling or directing them. However, the contemporary ethos is much more one of the professional as a member of a team, and beyond that, of an employing organisation. The presumption is that the individual professional will be subject to the rules, plans and priorities of that organisation. . . .

(Harrison and Pollitt 1994: 135; original emphasis)

Similarly, initiatives such as that concerning resource management could have far reaching effects upon both behaviour and values:

. . . a responsibility accounting system [such as RM] develops standards of behaviour such that 'normal' practice cannot only be defined, but also measured, and deviations noted. What is also implied is that what is rendered visible, measured, and rewarded gains legitimacy. Conversely, that which is not recognised by the formal system is often neither rewarded nor legitimate. . . .

(Bloomfield *et al.* 1992; cited in Latimer 1995: 217)

The colonising potential of such apparatuses is apparent in the argument that while nurses 'have reached . . . for managerialist devices to help them evidence (and some would assert, enhance) the effectiveness of their practices' (Latimer 1995: 217) they have run the risk of becoming redefined and controlled by such devices.

Johnson makes a similar point regarding the interrelation between government and the professions and the reproduction of expertise. He argues that the accepted understanding of the relationship between the state and the professions as one of a dichotomous tension between intervention and autonomy is misconceived (Johnson 1995). Drawing on Foucault's notion of governmentality – a collection of institutions, procedures, analyses and tactics that have characterised European government since the eighteenth and particularly nineteenth centuries (Foucault 1979) – he suggests that

expertise, as it became increasingly institutionalised in its professional form, became part of the process of governing. . . . There is a real sense in which in overseeing established definitions of illness, the profession is the state. . . . The expert is not sheltered by an environing state, but shares in the autonomy of the state.

(Johnson 1995: 8, 13)

Strengthening central surveillance and control

Since 1989 the NHS witnessed, as well as the introduction of the internal market which will be described shortly, a further tightening of the chain of management command running from the secretary of state down to district level. The government brought these changes about through the National Health Service and Community Care Act (1990). The scheme was set out in the White Paper, *Working for Patients* (Department of Health 1989c). District and regional health authorities were reconstituted as boards with executive and non-executive directors, the latter appointed by government ministers or regions: a 'purge' of local authority and professional representation, as one writer described it (Klein 1989: 239), demonstrating that such intermediary bodies were to become 'agents of the centre' (Wistow 1992: 109). Another commentator made a similar point:

> The NHS acquired a management culture of command and obedience more usually associated with private businesses than with public services in which those who failed to toe the policy line could be penalised in their career advancements and those who criticised it could place themselves at risk of disciplinary action.
>
> (Butler 1992: 36)

The policy of centralising control over decision-making while decentralising activity reflected a general trend in industry, a trend facilitated by the rise of information technology (IT) with its ability (in theory at least) to monitor from the centre performance at the periphery (Klein 1989). Pollitt has described the increased possibility for detailed day-to-day surveillance facilitated by this rise in IT as 'the information Panopticon' (Pollitt 1993: 117). The reader unfamiliar with Bentham's panopticon will find the scheme and its significance detailed in Chapter 2, pp. 9–11.

Hughes and Dingwall discuss the broad rhetorical context of the NHS reforms arguing that the 'motifs' of 'contract' and 'Trust' construct the changes and indeed the NHS itself as 'no more than an aggregate of individual decisions, while camouflaging great extensions to authoritarian power in the hands of the health secretary' (Hughes and Dingwall 1990). Kelly and Glover argue that the rhetoric of radical change within the NHS has been designed to conceal rather than to illuminate. In their view, the recent reforms do not mark a discontinuity with the past; rather they see the very inception of the NHS as guided by a modernist rationality which has simply been continuously developed. It was modernist for two main reasons: first, because of the belief that rational solutions could be found for organisational problems (and bureaucratic structures were one solution) and second, because of the assumption that the service's scientific expertise could be harnessed to effect a social engineering bringing about a national improvement in health (Kelly and Glover 1996). Within this overall continuity they see the Griffiths' reforms as a distinctive version. From 1948 to 1974 the governing rationality of the NHS had centred around attempts to improve bureaucratic efficiency. From 1983 new principles emerged in which financial efficiency became elevated from being one consideration among many to *the* major policy objective (ibid.: 20).

The 'internal market'

The creation of the so-called 'internal market', then, pushed the rationalisation of health care a further step. The central, neo-liberal, assumption behind *Working for Patients* was that if health care institutions were made to compete against each other within a market situation, this would result not only in greater efficiency but in improved responsiveness to its consumers (Harrison *et al.* 1990). The plan was said to owe much to the ideas of Enthoven (1985). It was brought into being by the separation of the *provision* of services (the employment of care delivery staff and ownership of health care institutions) from its *purchase*, or commission (the allocation of funds for provision to meet local population health needs). Institutions were enabled to apply to the secretary of state to become self-governing 'NHS Trusts'.

Advantages of such independence for Trusts included freedom from Whitley Council and other nationally agreed conditions of service for their employees and greater freedom in managing their own finances, such as the ability to borrow capital and accumulate surpluses for reinvestment. In 1991, 57 Trusts were established and 113 applications were made for the second wave in 1992, of which 99 were successful (Wistow 1992). By April 1993 there were 330 Trusts (Bartlett and Le Grand 1994) and by April 1994, when a further 143 hospitals and community units became Trusts, the total represented 96 per cent of hospital and community services (*HSJ News* 1994). The remaining 44 directly managed units were invited to apply for Trust status from April 1995 as part of the government's drive to complete the purchaser/provider split by that date. Similar moves occurred in Wales and Scotland (Shaw 1994: xviii).

As we have already seen (p. 38), the 1991 reforms involved two contradictory movements, a promise of autonomy at the same time as central control was increasing. What was spoken of as the final stage in a total restructuring of the health service was the amalgamation of the 14 regional health authorities (RHAs) into eight and their reconfiguration as outposts of the NHS Executive in 1996. From 1 April 1996 staff in the regional offices became civil servants, 'part of the centre rather than employees of a separate authority' with possible new dilemmas of loyalty (Stewart 1996).

Changes in primary care

The counterpart to the independence of Trust status in the primary care setting was the opportunity for general practitioners (GPs) with over 9,000 patients (7,000 from April 1993) to elect to become 'fundholders'. Fundholders receive a budget from their RHA which, in addition to contributions towards prescribing and staff salaries received by all GPs, contains an amount reflecting the practice's potential hospital referrals for certain procedures, based, initially, on its pre-application spending level. Corresponding amounts are deducted from the allocations of strategic authorities, i.e. district health authorities (DHAs). The commissioning responsibility of DHAs would thus steadily diminish as the number of fundholders increased (Butler 1992). First-wave GP fundholders came into existence on 1 April 1991, with each fundholder being awarded a special £16,000 start-up grant as well as a £33,000 annual management fee (Holliday 1992). During the course of this study, in April 1993, the scheme was extended. Fundholding GPs were given budgets to purchase district nursing and health visiting services from NHS community units. The guidelines expressly excluded the direct employment of community nurses. In April 1994 a further 850 GP practices joined the fundholding scheme, which meant that fundholders now had 36 per cent of the population on their lists (*HSJ News* 1994). A further extension of the fundholding scheme took place in that year enabling a wider range of GPs to join and further changes enabled 'single-handed' GPs to participate and extend fundholding to other areas of the budget. At the beginning of 1996, a total of 2,200 funds existed, approximately one practice in three in England. By April 1996 GP fundholders managed around 15 per cent of NHS spending on hospital and community services. At that time the membership of the National Association of Fundholding Practices stood at 1,050. During the first five years of fundholding, staff, equipment and computer costs of managing the scheme had cost £232 million. (*HSJ News Focus* 1996) as against £206 million efficiency savings (Audit Commission 1996a; 1996b).

Since the first days of fundholding and claims for its success (Brindle 1995), the Conservative government sought continually to expand the scheme. 'Total purchasing' pilot sites were established in which substantial increases in budget were offered to practices or 'multifunds' in order to purchase a complete range of health care services. Before the 1997 general election the Labour Party pledged to abolish fundholding in favour of locality purchasing where health authorities (the original purchasers of care), or the new commissioning agencies formed from the mergers of family health service authorities (FHSAs) with health authorities, would regain responsibility for purchasing local health care but seek the involvement of GPs through commissioning teams (Wainwright 1996). Before the election, the Conservative government placed continual emphasis on its desire to develop a 'primary care led NHS' focusing on new partnerships between health authorities, secondary care and local authorities, better team working with primary health care and the development of professional roles (Department of Health 1996a; Department of Health 1996b).

Managerialism

I have already described the strengthening of management controls introduced into the NHS but managerialism refers to a much deeper force felt on both sides of the Atlantic, not just in the public services. The following quotation suggests a useful definition of 'managerialism' as ideology:

> . . . the world should be a place where objectives are clear, where staff are highly motivated to achieve them, where close attention is given to monetary costs, where bureaucracy and red tape are eliminated. If one asks

how this is to be achieved the managerialist answer is, overwhelmingly, through the introduction of good management practices, which are assumed to be found at the highest pitch and most widely distributed in the private sector.

(Pollitt 1993: 7; original emphasis)

Some of the roots of managerialism might be located in the 'scientific management' advocated by American industrialist Frederick Winnslow Taylor at the beginning of this century. His starting-point was that 'the whole country is suffering through inefficiency'. The remedy lay in 'systematic management' which is 'a true science, resting upon clearly defined laws, rules and principles, as a foundation' (Taylor 1911). The principles which manifestly combine the modern characteristics of universality and impersonality, involve observation and measurement of output and the introduction of specific modifications such as rewards aimed at increasing worker performance (Kanigel 1997). Since then, however, successive sophistications, many associated with the influence of organisational and industrial psychologists, have entailed deeper penetrations into and attempts to control the consciousness of the worker (Pollitt 1993). The more recent of these involve motivational initiatives such as 'Total Quality Management', the growth of the management of 'human resources' and the rise of a discourse of 'organisational culture'.

Walby and Greenwell oppose two approaches to managerialism: Fordism, approximately the Taylorism referred to above, and post-Fordism, which has variously been termed 'new management' or human-resources management (Walby and Greenwell 1994). They consider these two approaches to be diametrically opposed in as far as Fordism can be characterised as the logic of tight control and post-Fordism as the fostering of self-motivation and autonomy among the workforce. These authors debate how far the NHS has seen a change in management style from one to the other. I will argue, however, that managerial talk of self-motivation, autonomy, excellence and closeness-to-the-customer can be understood as a rhetorical mask for the same Fordist drive for deep and penetrating control of the workforce by management (and ultimately by government). Walby and Greenwell present a predominantly task-orientated view of both the difference and the conflict between the nursing and medical professions, although, of course, they are aware of the immense institutional power base of medicine. They differentiate the impact of managerialism on the two occupations in terms of the relative autonomy of each. They view nursing as rigid, hierarchical and rule-bound and look to the 'extended role', i.e. carefully controlled situations where nurses may take on duties previously carried out by junior doctors, as an example of a newer move toward medical style individual judgement. However, it is important to be aware of the possibly different *rationalities* as well as rhetorics of the two professions and the fact that nurses may well construct their own version of autonomy characterised by moral agency and self-sacrifice. I will argue that this move characterises one mode of resistance to the power of managers.

Bureaucracies

Other roots of 'managerialism' can be traced to the growth of bureaucracies as a manifestation of modernity. Max Weber, writing in the early decades of the twentieth century, offered the most well-known early studies of this phenomenon which have given rise to a considerable body of literature. Celia Davies has recently examined some of this literature and its particular application to nurses working as professionals within bureaucracies (Davies 1995). She focuses on how bureaucracy (as well as professionalism to which it is often opposed) can be understood as having an implicit male gendering. She does this by examining how Weber's early work singled out key features of bureaucracy: impartiality of decision-making, the impersonality of the bureaucrat and the authoritative character of hierarchy, and then linking these attributes to those that are said to characterise 'male' approaches to problem-solving and interaction (Chodorow 1978; Gilligan 1982).

Although it is possible to criticise the universalising tendencies of the claims of the writers on which Davies bases this view of gendering (Fraser and Nicholson 1990), her theory can be usefully applied to any study of management. Of particular relevance to the present project is the understanding of managerial rationality that Davies offers. She draws out the acontextual basis of bureaucratic decision-making: 'Formality and distance are not only valued, but are seen as the only route to a rational decision' (Davies 1995: 53). However, drawing on the work of Pringle (1988) with secretaries, she suggests that '[w]e must understand "ordered rationality" as an illusion' (Davies 1995: 55). This is because women in organisations are continually but invisibly carrying out a range of facilitating work that would not meet the criteria of rationality yet without which organisations would be unable to function and male managers would not be able to continue to act in 'disembodied' ways. She suggests that there are alternative modes of rationality that are difficult to articulate because they have been culturally assigned to femininity. Although it appears that this 'distant' model of managing and management does not sit comfortably with contemporary 'cultural' management like that advocated by Peters and Waterman (1982), she argues that the new manager has, in fact, many of the characteristics of the old: 'He takes a critical stance towards the arguments and established practices of others, asking continually for outcome data, cost information and performance measures' (Davies 1995: 168–169).

The 'new management' operates under a 'different mantle of neutrality' (Gray and Jenkins 1993) and takes a 'retreat into technique' (Harrison *et al.* 1992) that masks the transposition of political questions into scientific and technical issues. Although such rhetoric was indeed offered by the managers involved in this study, along with the intense scrutiny of outcome data and cost information mentioned above, such a commentary does not account for these managers' talk of a strong commitment to providing health care to their local population.

Contrary to what Davies and others have argued, the managers in the present study spoke of being engaged in a moral activity and a pragmatic struggle between operationalising explicit values and working within reduced resource levels. Their approaches, or at least their own descriptions of their approaches, involved cunning and imagination alongside, or intermingled with, the 'neutral' mechanisms of measurement and cost control. If their espousal of values – other than the values of effectiveness – was not merely a *conscious* and cynical rhetorical front, we need to look in more detail if we are to develop our descriptions of contemporary health care management. The deconstructive approach offered in this book facilitates a sensitivity to such discourse. It provides an understanding of the almost independent life of the text and the way it provides a space for the subjectivity of those caught up within it. Certain language is so available to health service managers that they almost cannot help but adopt it.

Bureaucracy and morality

MacIntyre (1985) writes about Weber's view of bureaucracy and the contemporary manager from a moral perspective. He argues initially that we live in the aftermath of the failure of the Enlightenment's project to justify and ground morality by appeals to reason and rationality (utilitarianism he argues was one such failure). In our age and culture, moral judgements have become nothing but expressions of preference, of attitude or feeling masquerading as universal statements. Consequently all moral disagreements have become rationally interminable because they typically involve protagonists who do not share a moral frame of reference. However, MacIntyre is careful not to universalise this fragmented situation and contrasts his own view with a range of philosophers and other thinkers who have made this very universalising mistake. He terms the universalising of this position *emotivism*:

> What I have suggested to be the case by and large about our own culture – that in moral argument the apparent assertion of principles functions as a mask for expressions of personal preference – is what emotivism takes to be universally the case.
>
> (ibid.: 19)

MacIntyre's second point concerns the issue of persuasion and manipulation. Because we have no unassailable criteria from which to make up our own minds about moral action, we are faced with a dilemma when we wish to recommend or request action from others. He suggests that those attempting to persuade others to carry out particular courses of action have two different approaches at their disposal. First, they can use personal, if inadequate, criteria: 'Do this because I wish it.' In this instance whether these are sufficient criteria to persuade the hearer to act depends upon a range of personal and contextual factors, for example whether the person making the utterance is in a position of authority over the other. Or second, and MacIntyre argues that this is characteristic of our culture and times, the speaker can appeal to purportedly impersonal rational criteria: 'Do this because it is your duty' or 'Do this because it would give pleasure to a number of people', or, extending his notion to the circumstances of the present study, 'Do this because it is the most efficient use of fixed resources.'

For MacIntyre, Weber was both an emotivist and one who dealt at length with notions of power and authority. Questions about ends, according to MacIntyre were for Weber questions about values, and reason, according to emotivists, has nothing to say about values. For Weber, each individual's conscience is irrefutable and choices about values rest upon purely subjective judgements (MacIntyre 1985). As a consequence of this position, Weber's distinction between power and authority on the grounds that authority legitimately serves particular ends and faiths, is thus untenable because no type of authority can appeal to any rational criteria 'except that kind of bureaucratic authority which appeals precisely to its own *effectiveness*' (ibid.: 26; original emphasis). In other words bureaucratic authority is nothing other than successful power. Sociologists since Weber, even while attempting to shift the focus of the study of managerial action from those issues emphasised by him, have tended to reinforce his account by looking at, for example, managers' need to influence the motives of their subordinates or to ensure that those subordinates argue from premises that support their own prior conclusions (Likert 1961; cited in MacIntyre 1985: 27). On a Weberian reading then, the modern manager represents the obliteration of the distinction between manipulative and non-manipulative social relations. We will return to MacIntyre's critique of the authority of the contemporary manager in Chapter 9.

In the present project I examine issues of persuasion and manipulation as they are effected through language. Ricoeur, in a linguistic and semantic study of metaphor, reminds us that metaphor 'redescribes' reality (Ricoeur 1986: 22) and summarises Aristotelian and Platonic suspicion of rhetoric:

> The technique founded on knowledge of the factors that help to effect persuasion puts formidable power in the hands of anyone who masters it perfectly – the power to manipulate words apart from things, and to manipulate men by manipulating words.
>
> (ibid.: 11)

The issue of manipulation and the redescription of reality through rhetoric is apparent in the attention to organisational culture that has gained ascendancy in managerial literature and which, in the last decade, entered NHS managerial discourse (Pollitt 1991). It has also, as we shall soon see, entered nursing's own discourse at a national level.

The new addition: cultural control

While not supplanting the continuing emphasis on economy and efficiency, this new drive adds to it notions such as 'cultural change' and 'quality' both borrowed from the private sector, notions with which it may have been hoped to 'rescue the sagging morale of public service staff' and 'rehabilitate the Government's reputation as caring for the public services' (Harrison and Pollitt 1994). Initiatives like the *Citizen's Charter* and a number of further charters devised in its wake signalled the government's attention to, at least the rhetoric of, quality public services. Perhaps more significantly, the successful marketing to managers of the notion of 'organisational culture' borrowed from sociology and anthropology in, perhaps, a 'crude and excessively plastic manner' (Ferlie 1997: 184), accounted for its spread into the public sector. The ultimate end, however, is instrumental, that is, increased organisational performance or increased market share or commercial survival, and its chief assumption is that those who run the organisation are the most appropriate people to determine the organisation's culture. In the present study, as will be shown, one manager explicitly, and almost every other manager implicitly, paid allegiance to these notions. Harrison and Pollitt draw attention to the colonising power of such an approach by the juxtaposition of two quotations:

> Psychologists study the need for self-determination in a field called 'illusion of control'. Simply stated, its findings indicate that if people think they have even modest personal control over their destinies, they will persist at tasks. They will do better at them. They will become more committed to them. . . . The fact . . . that we *think* we have a *bit* more discretion leads to *much* greater commitment.
>
> (Peters and Waterman 1982: 80–81: original italics)

> Is it not the supreme and most insidious exercise of power to prevent people, to whatever degree, from having grievances by shaping their perceptions, cognitions and preferences in such a way that they accept their role in the existing order of things, either because they see it as natural and unchangeable, or because they value it as divinely organised and beneficial?
>
> (Lukes 1994: 24)

Pollitt (1993: 114) critiques the political New Right's commitment to managerialism and its possible dangers. In quoting Winner, the location of managerialism within both a growing social movement and a distinctively modern, universalising project is beginning to be made clear:

> Efficiency, speed, precise measurement, rationality, productivity, and technical improvement become ends in themselves, applied obsessively to areas in life in which they would previously have been rejected as inappropriate. Efficiency – the quest for maximum output per unit – is, no one would question, of paramount importance in technical systems. But now efficiency takes on a more general value and becomes a universal maxim for all intelligent conduct.
>
> (Winner 1977: 299)

Phenomena such as the increasing possibilities for highly technological and costly medical interventions within a cost-constrained situation, the rise in numbers of the elderly population, 'rationing' issues, attempts to democratise this process and the rise of health economics seem likely to intensify any government's and any management team's attention to issues of efficiency within a health service.

THE ORIGINAL RESEARCH

In mid- to late 1990, research was being planned at the Royal College of Nursing (RCN) as a response to the NHS changes that had been announced in January of the previous year. The aim was to 'document and analyse the impact of legislative and organisational change on the organisation and morale of nurses working in a selection of community trusts' (Wade 1991: 10). The methods were to be twofold: the measurement of nurses' job satisfaction using a questionnaire, and semi-structured interviews carried out with all levels of manager in four of the new first wave NHS Trusts that operated in a community setting. The purpose of the interviews was to discover 'strategies' adopted by managers in response to the legislative changes. The Trusts chosen were the first to grant full permission to proceed and the research was to continue over the first three years of their operation. This would enable changes in both job satisfaction and strategy to be described, and the two, possibly, to be linked. Also it would be possible to compare the relative satisfaction of different groups of nurse, for example nurses based in GP practices and health visitors. The community setting was chosen partly because additional legislation was planned for that area of health care (Department of Health 1989a) and partly because of the research unit's commitment to working in that setting. Confidential reports of satisfaction would be made available to the managers and nurses themselves in each Trust. It was after the management of one of the Trusts had read the first report that it announced its decision to withdraw from the research. This action, along with the tense meeting between research staff and two personnel managers and a senior nurse manager from the Trust, provided as eloquent an account of 'strategy' as any interview. The Trust's managers suggested that this research, with its RCN connection, had a 'hidden agenda' to attack Trusts. (Further details of the research interviews are provided in Chapter 5).

As well as this unforeseen turn, the research ran longer than planned because the start of the interviews with managers was delayed. Yearly reports of its findings (Traynor and Wade 1992; Traynor 1993; Traynor and Wade 1994; Traynor 1995) were produced and sometimes drawn upon by the RCN in its various pay campaigns and to use as evidence (Royal College of Nursing 1995).

In this book I will develop some of the ideas only touched upon in the RCN research. I hope to bring what was marginal in that research (such as nurses' textual comments) to the centre and displace its central concerns (organisational details) and approaches (attempts to measure job satisfaction) to the periphery.

THE STRUCTURE OF THIS BOOK

The next chapter describes the epistemological atmosphere within which this work gradually developed by examining the influence of 'postmodernism', chiefly through the works of four of its major figures. It also extracts from their writing concerns that are developed in this book: those of knowledge, power and their intimate connection. The confidence with which knowledge claims can be made, including those made throughout the book, is undercut. A brief background to 'modernism' is also given for those readers who require it.

The approaches to the texts I have attempted to use, namely, 'deconstruction' brought to prominence by French philosopher and literary theorist Jacques Derrida and certain approaches to discourse analysis are focused on in Chapter 3. This is prefaced by a short history of the way in which the boundaries between certain academic disciplines have been disrupted. These include the traditional areas of philosophy, literary criticism and social theory. This work is located at the peripheries of (at least) these three disciplines.

Chapter 4 attempts to locate some of the writing of nursing's leaders within the 'discourses of the Enlightenment' and to identify a range of professionalising endeavours as a distinctively modern project. It draws in nursing's response to the rise of evidence-based health care. It also suggests a 'deontological' (Seedhouse 1993) context for other voices within the nursing profession, particularly those of individual care givers such as those involved in this research.

The details of the research study including descriptions of the sample, study design, data collection and time span are given in Chapter 5. A fuller account is also given of how the interview transcripts and questionnaire comments are approached as 'texts'.

Chapters 6 and 7 apply the textual approaches introduced in Chapter 3 to examine the texts of the interviews with health service managers, while the written and spoken comments of nurses involved in care delivery are presented in Chapter 8.

Chapter 9 offers a reflection on whether the book's exploration of the texts of nurses and managers has let us think in new ways about profession and power, organisation(s) and power, subjectivity/identity and the project of inquiry itself.

2 Sawing off the branch and sitting: the context of the postmodern

INTRODUCTION

Since the appearance of the term, initially in architecture and soon after in philosophy and social theory, postmodernism has had a brilliant career, emerging now somewhat battered at the end of the 1990s. It has been condemned as faddish, condoning political conservatism, a self-indulgent past-time of a disenchanted intellectual elite. Bruno Latour, for one, can find no words 'ugly enough to designate this intellectual movement – or rather this intellectual immobility' (Latour 1993: 61). Its kindred terms, deconstruction and post-structuralism, have fared little better, the discovery of the anti-Semitic wartime writing of Belgian literary theorist Paul de Man providing, for those eager to discredit deconstruction, powerful evidence of its moral bankruptcy (Norris 1990a). Post-structuralism has been described as a cynical invention on the part of French intellectuals like Michel Foucault to maintain reputation and position in post-1968 Paris when student rebellion turned against the established intellectual hegemony of, among other teachings, structuralism (Turner 1994).

Postmodernism has become simultaneously controversial and, in the arguments of many, a straw figure, a latter-day positivism, more of a collection of caricature positions to be blown down in the service of various projects. Of course, critics have grappled with postmodernism's content and its implications, arguing against what they see as its self-contradiction and lack of critical force. There has been disagreement among those figures seen as its major voices. However, at the same time many of its insights, or the insights that it has articulated, have become common currency in social theory and literary criticism – the linking of power and knowledge, the denial of the possibility of a context-free knowledge that rises above language, an exposing of metaphysical first principles as smuggled into an argument from within a contingent scheme. In this sense, postmodernism and these other intellectual movements have won the day. Yet however pleased we may be about this Pyrrhic victory, we could well be left with a champion without much appetite for 'real' fights, against social inequalities and oppression for instance. I will try to argue the case for the usefulness of 'postmodern research' in the last chapter but I must leave the reader to judge whether the whole project of this book has contributed to an erosion of the credibility and power of the force of managerialism.

Postmodernism plays two central roles in this work. First, it provides a powerful critique of epistemology and methodology, demanding that the process of inquiry itself be drastically recast. The notion of representing reality, of holding the mirror up to nature, of discovering the truth of the situation is abandoned as a mirage. In its place is an understanding of inquiry as a recontextualising of beliefs. In place of the metaphor of convergence upon truth is the notion of proliferation, of diversity rather than unity.

Second, postmodernism also provides an approach to the plurality of discourses within health care in the NHS of the late 1990s. It offers approaches to the history of how a particular discourse has become dominant; it draws us in to the project of detailing the mechanisms of this domination and colonisation of other non-legitimated discourses.

After evoking something of the context from which postmodernism has emerged, in this chapter I will discuss the work of four writers who have been described as being responsible for 'mainstream postmodernist theory': Jean François Lyotard, Richard Rorty, Michel Foucault and Jacques Derrida (Di Stefano 1987; cited in Harding 1990). It is these writers' questioning of the authority and effects of reason and their linking of these effects with the controlling regimes of powerful groups that makes an understanding of their work essential for this examination of the power of both managerialism and professionalism. It is into this theoretical context that the texts of both managers and nurses will be placed.

Post-what? Modernity?

The reign of what has come to be known as 'modernity' finds its origin partly with the work of astronomical geniuses of the sixteenth and seventeenth centuries and partly with European philosophers such as Descartes, Hume and Kant, who, each in their different ways gave the astronomers' methods – whether observation or rational thought or a combination of the two – the metaphysical privilege of being able to discover the secrets of humankind and the universe. Such a privileging of method, though useful, can be held up to question.

Bertrand Russell, writing in the 1940s, considered that 'The modern world, so far as mental outlook is concerned, begins in the seventeenth century' (Russell 1991).

Science

Scientists, among them the astronomers, Copernicus, Kepler, Galileo and Newton, self-consciously developed a new method for discovering knowledge and in the process laid foundations for a new epistemology. They stressed meticulous observation, empirical demonstration and a scepticism towards previous explanations for events that might be superficial, superstitious and wrong. These scientific advances took place in astronomy and mathematics and the two were closely interrelated. This is the period of the invention of a number of important scientific instruments including the telescope and the microscope, instruments that facilitated an accelerating range of discoveries. It was also a period of decisive advance in mathematics especially by Newton and Galileo. Observation, coupled with mathematical calculation, gave modern science its new ability to predict events. Scientists now proposed 'laws' such as Newton's laws of motion. Newton's law of universal gravitation, for example, at once made everything in planetary theory deducible.

The question of authority was central to the controversies that astronomers such as Copernicus and Galileo experienced with the Church (both Catholic and Protestant). Calvin is said to have exclaimed 'Who will venture to place the authority of Copernicus above that of the Holy Spirit?' (Russell 1991: 515). A central characteristic, therefore, of modernity is that it offered a new authority of observation and measurement, an authority of method over the authority of tradition and revelation.

The influence of science on philosophy

If the basic processes of nature involved regular, predictable motion, mused seventeenth-century philosophers, human behaviour might also be described in mechanical and dynamic terms rather than in terms of the moral free will, or the teleology of earlier thinkers. Although humankind may have been removed from a place at the apex of God's creation to a more humble position, the achievement of explaining and predicting the movement of heavenly bodies more than compensated.

Humanity itself and human nature soon came to be described as mechanical systems, the circulation of the blood around the body, revealed by Harvey in 1628, mirroring the regular predictable movement of the stars. Metaphysical causes and purposes were erased from the rhetoric of scientific enquiry although it is possible to argue, as Kant did, that the assumption of regularity itself is tantamount to a metaphysics. To summarise, observation and mathematics were seen as offering the key to the discoveries of nature. According to Russell: 'The reign of law had established its hold on men's imagination, making such things as magic and sorcery incredible' (Russell 1991: 522).

So we enter this period, in seventeenth- and eighteenth-century Europe (particularly in France and Scotland) known as the Enlightenment, the Age of Reason. It is a period characterised by a belief that the use of reason and rationality offers the key to social progress and human destiny. This philosophical and cultural vitality was laid upon the foundations of optimism and humanistic boldness that the significant developments of the physical sciences provided. Perhaps always hand in hand with science, the Enlightenment's influence can be seen in the triumphalism of the industrial revolution of the eighteenth and nineteenth centuries. Its far-reaching effects have been subject to fierce attack by Adorno and Horkheimer in *Dialectic of Enlightenment* (Adorno and Horkheimer 1979).

Enlightenment and scholarship

Prior to the Enlightenment, the task of scholarship was seen as one of revealing the word of God as manifest in creation. The notion of seeking the 'God's-eye view', the view free from the perspectives of particular individuals or groups, endured the increasing marginalisation of the Creator. Although other ideals, such as historicism, hermeneutics and perhaps phenomenology, and traditions have surfaced in the wake of the Kantian belief in the subjective origin of the organising principles of the universe, the approach of objectivism can be seen to have dominated natural and social sciences and philosophy which has been considered as 'the elaborator of those basic principles by which all claims to knowledge were to be judged' (Nicholson 1990: 2). Allegiance to the norm of objectivity stands as its testimony. The search for universal laws found its place within the study of human nature and society and by the end of the eighteenth century its mode of knowledge came to be grounded, in England and France, in empiricist and rationalist epistemologies (Seidman and Wagner 1992: 3). With this was linked the conviction that scientific enlightenment would act as a force of social progress, enabling humanity to emerge from prejudice and ignorance. This ambition formed the basis for the emergence of sociology in the nineteenth century. It has particularly become associated with positivism and its twentieth-century re-emergence as the logical positivism of the Vienna circle (Stumpf 1993).

A number of groups have criticised the norm of objectivity and the alleged neutrality of the scholarly endeavour. Feminists, as well as those involved in the gay and black liberation movements, have argued that what had often been presented as objective and free from the influence of values, such as those related to gender, had actually reflected those values. Claiming that such biases were inevitable, they contended that all scholarship reflected the perspectives and ideals of its originators. Before postmodernism, the so-called masters of suspicion, Freud, Marx and Nietzsche, undermined both the transparency of the human spectator subject and the domination implicit in Western rationality with, since Plato, its dualism of appearance and reality and programme of advancing conceptual thought at the expense of the heterogeneity of material (Benhabib 1990: 110–111).

The postmodernist critique focuses on the very criteria by which claims of knowledge are legitimised, arguing that the criteria by which the true is distinguished from the false cannot themselves be legitimised outside the traditions of modernity and that they have become the means for the exercise of power in an ever-widening domain. These criteria that separate science from superstition and myth – legitimate knowledge from what Foucault calls 'low-ranking . . . unqualified, even directly disqualified knowledges' (Foucault 1980b: 82) – become the taken-for-granted foundation for a range of activities undertaken by natural and social scientists and others who see their work as inspired by science. Within philosophy, writers such as Richard Rorty critique the very notion of a theory of knowledge, arguing that the quest for such a theory rests upon the modernist notion of a transcendental reason, a reason independent not only of history and location but also of the body.

There is diversity within the writing of the authors described as postmodern but they share certain tendencies, certain moves: a turning away from universal justifications or foundations for knowledge toward local, contingent knowledges shared by communities without claim to any metaphysical foundation. They explore both the implications of such a move for the process of inquiry, for example within the natural and human sciences and in philosophy, and the political implications for society as a whole. They seek to make explicit the relationship between claims to having access to knowledge and power and tell the history of such power relationships. They are interested in investigating local phenomena and difference rather than aiming for grand explanation. They have a tendency to break down or *deconstruct* well-established boundaries, for example that between philosophy and literary criticism and dualisms, such as that between cause and effect, and to explore alternative, previously metaphorical or marginal readings of familiar texts, histories and phenomena. In describing these characteristics, I have summarised my approach within this book.

The *locus classicus* for the postmodern debate is Jean-François Lyotard's *The Postmodern Condition: A Report on Knowledge* published in 1979. His work is of particular interest drawing out as it does differences between 'scientific' and 'narrative' knowledge that find certain parallels in the talk of managers and nurses in this study.

THE DEATH OF THE GRAND NARRATIVE

For Lyotard, postmodernism describes a general condition of Western civilisation, a civilisation within which the legitimising grand narratives or meta-narratives behind social and scientific theorising have lost, or are in the process of losing, credibility:

> Science has always been in conflict with narratives. Judged by the yardstick of science, the majority of them prove to be fables. But to the extent that science does not restrict itself to stating useful regularities and seeks the truth, it is obliged to legitimate the rules of its own game. It then produces a discourse of legitimation with respect to its own status, a discourse called philosophy. I will use the term *modern* to designate any science that legitimates itself with reference to a metadiscourse of this kind making an explicit appeal to some grand narrative, such as the dialectics of Spirit, the hermeneutics of meaning, the emancipation of the rational or working subject, or the creation of wealth.
>
> (Lyotard 1979: xxiii; original emphasis)

Narrative knowledge, for its part, appears to need little legitimation:

> Narrative knowledge does not give priority to the question of its own
> legitimation and . . . it certifies itself in the pragmatics of its own trans-
> mission without having recourse to argumentation and proof.
>
> (Lyotard 1979: 27)

In the place of a privileged discourse that can situate and evaluate all other
discourses without itself being infected by historicity and contingency (Fraser
and Nicholson 1990) has come an era of plurality, locality and contingency.
Even in scientific inquiry, Lyotard argues, the metaphysical quest for a first
proof and transcendental authority has given way to an acknowledgement that
the 'rules of the game of science' can only be legitimated within a debate that
is already scientific in nature. In other words, it is only scientific consensus
that deems these rules good. So how does Lyotard describe the activities of
science and theorising in general? He sees scientific and narrative knowledges,
their relationship and much of social relations, in terms of *language games* – a
term he borrows from Wittgenstein in which utterances can be described in
terms of rules specifying their properties and the uses to which they can be
put – as with pieces in a game of chess. Also like game playing, 'speech acts'
involve us in *agonistics*, contests. Science is concerned primarily with denotive
statements and, for Lyotard, science is a subset of learning which is in itself
a subset of knowledge. Knowledge is not comprised of a set of denotive
statements but rather of wide-ranging notions like *savoir-faire*, *savoir-vivre*,
savoir-écouter (know how, knowing how to live, knowing how to listen).
Knowledge enables its possessor to form 'good' utterances be they denotive,
prescriptive or evaluative. Such utterances are judged to be 'good' when they
conform to the relevant criteria accepted in the social circle with whom the
'knower' converses.

> The early philosophers called this mode of legitimating statements opinion.
> The consensus that permits such knowledge to be circumscribed and makes
> it possible to distinguish one who knows from one who doesn't (the
> foreigner, the child) is what constitutes the culture of a people.
>
> (Lyotard 1979: 19)

Lyotard goes on to say,

> Drawing a parallel between science and nonscientific (narrative) knowledge
> helps us understand, or at least sense, that the former's existence is no more
> – and no less – necessary than the latter's. Both are composed of sets of
> statements; the statements are 'moves' made by the players within the
> framework of generally applicable rules; these rules are specific to each
> particular kind of knowledge, and the 'moves' judged to be 'good' in one
> cannot be of the same type as those judged 'good' in another, unless it
> happens that way by chance.
>
> (ibid.: 26)

However, the relationship between narrative and scientific discourse has been far from harmonious. If narrative knowledge is tolerant towards science, modern science does not share the same liberality. The modern scientist concludes that narrative statements lack validity because of the absence of argumentation or proof. This demand for legitimation has characterised the history of Western cultural imperialism classifying narrative knowledge as 'underdeveloped, backward, alienated, composed of opinions, customs, authority, prejudice, ignorance, ideology . . . fit only for women and children' (Lyotard 1979: 27). This epistemological imperialism, I will argue, is apparent in the participating managers' estimation of the views of sections of their nursing workforce. By way of contrast *post*modern science, having experienced quantum mechanics, microphysics, chaos and catastrophe theories is 'theorising its own evolution as discontinuous, catastrophic, nonrectifiable, and paradoxical. It is changing the meaning of the word knowledge, while expressing how such a change can take place' (ibid.: 60).

The dominant move in postmodern science, argues Lyotard, is not consensus but dissension, a continual destabilising of the existing paradigm. Consensus can be understood not as the unforced agreement of knowing intellects in dialogue but as a component of a particular system that is manipulated by that system in order to improve its performance. The ultimate goal within this description is power. It is because of this that some scientists have seen their new move ignored or repressed because it too abruptly destabilises accepted positions within the institution of power. Lyotard deems such repressive activity 'terrorism'. It occurs wherever players are silenced or consent, not because their argument has been refuted but because their ability to participate has been threatened. It is a characteristic of 'institutions of knowledge' and 'decision makers' rather than of science itself; indeed, the pragmatics of science where a statement is considered worth retaining when it marks a difference from what is already known, makes science an 'antimodel of a stable system' (Lyotard 1979: 64).

But if there has been a growing incredulity towards metanarratives then 'the system' (political or institutional) seeking the totality with which Lyotard urges us to make war has endeavoured to replace it with the criterion of performance and efficiency. It is because of this that he suggests the search for universal consensus, urged by Habermas (1984), is both naive and dangerous. Behind such a view he detects two assumptions; that it is possible that all speakers could come to agreement on universal rules valid for all language games and that the ultimate goal of dialogue is consensus, whereas, according to his analysis of science, consensus is only a particular state of discussion rather than its end. 'Consensus has become an outmoded and suspect value' (Lyotard 1979: 66). He suggests a way out of this impasse. What is needed instead, is to arrive at a justice that is not linked to notions of universal consensus. 'The only "we" we need is a local and temporary one', agrees Rorty, commenting on Lyotard's thought (Rorty 1991a: 214). Lyotard proposes a plurality of local, always provisional, agreements on prescriptives for language games, a condition of 'temporary contract' that he believes is already replacing permanent institutions within 'the professional, emotional, sexual, cultural, family, and international domains' (Lyotard 1979: 66). The 'system', with its single criterion of performativity, may view this ambivalently; on the one hand, plurality makes totality harder to achieve but on the other, a certain flexibility can lead to creative turmoil and increased operativity. Ambivalent too is the role of increasing computerisation within society. From the system's point of view the computer could be the 'dream machine' of ultimate control but Lyotard's democratic alternative could 'give the public free access to the memory and data banks' in which case language games would be games 'of perfect information at any moment'. In these games, Lyotard concludes his essay:

> . . . the stakes would be Knowledge (or information, if you will), and the reserve of knowledge – language's reserve of possible utterances – is inexhaustible. This sketches the outline of a politics that would respect both the desire for justice and the desire for the unknown.
>
> (ibid: 67)

From the evidence of this study, however, there is little to suggest that computers offer a source of democracy within the institutions under study.

Such writing disrupts the authority of knowledge claims, leaving any investigation, such as this one, in a precarious position. Is it dangerous to take up the arguments of postmodernism if we wish to say anything we want listened to? I will be discussing this dilemma in Chapter 9.

OBJECTIVITY, REPRESENTATION AND THE PROCESS OF INQUIRY

Richard Rorty's notions of inquiry and truth, I suggest, let us saw off the branch we are sitting on (my words) while still allowing us to make admirable sense of our lives (his words).

Rorty urges us to abandon the notion of human inquiry, and philosophy in particular, as representation of an external reality. Inquiry is not a matter of 'getting reality right' or rising out of *local* language into neutral or *real* language; in other words getting a God's-eye view. For him, inquiry is rather the reweaving of a web of beliefs in the light of new, puzzling stimuli. Like both Lyotard and Foucault, Rorty is aware of the unavoidable link between knowledge and power:

> . . . any academic discipline which wants a place at the trough, but is unable to offer the predictions and the technology provided by the natural sciences, must either pretend to imitate science or find some way of obtaining 'cognitive status' without the necessity of discovering facts.
>
> (Rorty 1991c: 35)

Rorty abandons notions of objectivity and subjectivity in favour of the idea of greater or lesser degrees of unforced agreement. He describes the representationalist search for Truth as characterised by appeals to natural or universal rather than local criteria. For the representationalist, there is a notion of convergence about truth; truth is 'out there' awaiting discovery and more or less accurate representation. Rorty offers instead an idea of inquiry as proliferating rather than converging, giving rise to diversity rather than unity. Within his notion of inquiry there is no privileging of explanation over and above interpretation. In fact, he argues, there is no useful distinction between these two terms and no distinction between objects constituted by language and those which are not. For him, all are. He argues that once we rid ourselves of the idea of different methods appropriate to the natures of different objects, we give our attention instead to questions concerning the purpose which a particular inquiry is supposed to serve and value different tools for different tasks (Rorty 1989).

Rorty goes on to identify two groups: 'realists' – those who wish to ground a desire for solidarity in objectivity and devise an epistemology which makes possible a natural and not merely social justification for beliefs, and 'pragmatists' who wish to reduce objectivity to solidarity. For realists, truth is the result of the application of those 'genuinely' rational procedures of justification, correspondence to reality, to the intrinsic nature of things. Pragmatists view truth as 'what it is good for us to believe' and do not require a correspondent account of the relationship between beliefs and objects:

> From a pragmatist point of view, to say that what is rational for us now to believe may not be *true*, is simply to say that somebody may come up with a better idea. It is to say that there is always room for improved belief, since new evidence, or a new hypothesis, or a whole new vocabulary, may come along.
>
> (Rorty 1991d: 23; original emphasis)

A number of consequences follow from the pragmatist's decision to abandon epistemological groundings for inquiry, for culture, or for any area of human activity. One is that the link between culture and knowledge, or rather, widely accepted procedures for justification, becomes more apparent:

> I think that putting the issue [of relativism] in such moral and political terms, rather than epistemological or metaphysical terms, makes clearer what is at stake. For now the question is not about how to define words like 'truth' or 'rationality' or 'knowledge' or 'philosophy', but about what self-image our society should have of itself. The ritual invocation of the 'need to avoid relativism' is most comprehensible as an expression of the need to preserve certain habits of contemporary European life. These are the habits nurtured by the Enlightenment, and justified by it in terms of an appeal of Reason, conceived as a transcultural human ability to correspond to reality,

a faculty whose possession and use is demonstrated by obedience to explicit criteria.

(Rorty 1991d: 28)

Another consequence is that it is possible to value institutions and practices such as those of science or religion, or notions such as liberalism, but at the same time reject their metaphysical groundings, and propose instead a better non-metaphysical grounding. Rorty explains the privileged (in both senses) position given to science as a cultural lag that allowed an older religious language and aspiration to be attached to the emergent natural sciences during the Enlightenment.

Communication with others

If Rorty rejects an ahistorical touchstone of truth located outside culture to which appeals can be made to settle disputes between groups – and such appeals were made both by nurses and by managers in this study – how then can these different groups communicate or, to use Rorty's example, on what grounds can liberals criticise or express outrage at Nazism? This is a central dilemma in this research. Rorty uses the term ethnocentric to convey his belief that communities can only work by their own lights. He argues that realists are just as ethnocentric as pragmatists but that realists draw comfort from universalising their own culture's values and aspirations in a way that pragmatists do not; the ideal human society will always look suspiciously like the one *we* identify with.

> I have been arguing that we pragmatists should grasp the ethnocentric horn of this dilemma. We should say that we must, in practice, privilege our own group, even though there can be no noncircular justification for doing so. We must insist that the fact that nothing is immune from criticism does not mean that we have a duty to justify everything. We Western liberal intellectuals should accept the fact that we have to start from where we are, and that there are lots of views which we simply cannot take seriously.
>
> (Rorty 1991d: 29)

All we can do is to argue, albeit passionately, from our own community's point of view, without claiming or aiming for objectivity. Often, there are enough shared beliefs for dialogue to take place between different communities. In this situation we may attempt to justify our beliefs to others whose beliefs overlap ours to some appropriate extent, but conversion to or from another point of view will not be a matter of inference from previously shared premises. It is unhelpful, he argues, to be 'scientific' about our moral and political lives.

Being scientific, before Kuhn, was a matter of staying within a logical space which forms an intrinsically privileged context. Rorty suggests that although 'enlightened post-Kuhnians' may be free from this notion, they have yet to escape the idea that inquiry is a matter of 'finding out the nature of something which lies outside the web of beliefs and desires. There still lingers some sense in which the object of inquiry . . . has a context of its own, a context which is privileged by virtue of it being the object's rather than the enquirer's' (Rorty 1991b: 96). The pragmatist's position, as formulated by Rorty, recognises a relation of *causation* between beliefs and other items in the universe but not one of *representation*. Beliefs may be *about* nonbeliefs but only in a loose sense; the sense in which, for example, Shakespeare's play is *about* Hamlet. Aboutness is not a matter of pointing outside the web of beliefs but of drawing attention to beliefs relevant to the justification of other beliefs.

In reply to questions about objects and their contexts, Rorty's pragmatist claims that all objects are always already contextualised. They all come with contexts attached. He rejects claims that sociology differs from the natural sciences in that it deals with a pre-interpreted world and that everyday experience, because it is already symbolically structured, is inaccessible to 'mere observation'. Rorty suggests that it is because of the very 'theory-dependency of data description' spoken about by Habermas (1984: 110) that the notion of 'mere observation' is *equally* redundant in the natural and social sciences. Once this long-standing opposition between context and thing contextualised is dropped, it is no longer possible to divide the universe up into things with intrinsic properties or natures and things which are dependent on context for what they are, or as Rorty put it, to make a distinction between 'hard lumps and squishy texts' (Rorty 1991b).

In response to the attack that this understanding of inquiry means that the inquirer never gets outside their own head, Rorty argues that all anybody can do is to reweave a web of beliefs in the light of new stimuli. However, this is not as bad as it might sound (to realists) as anti-essentialists admit that objects they do not control cause them to change their beliefs, sometimes drastically, with the result that he or 'she is no more free from pressure from outside, no more tempted to be arbitrary than anyone else' (Rorty 1991b: 101). He or she may be free from the concern for representing things as they *really, intrinsically* are, but not from the need to fit in unexpected events into the rest of his or her beliefs.

One implication of adopting an anti-essentialist view is the belief that *all* inquiry is recontextualisation. The distinction between interpretation and the supposedly harder, more reliable, explanation, disappears. From this, in turn, would follow the belief that the only difference between sociologists and physicists would be a sociological one, not a methodological or philosophical one. Rorty argues that even objects which we might consider reassuringly solid and free of symbolic meaning may well turn out to be very different entities; such as the rabbits that were, according to Quine, worshipped by the inhabitants of one particular culture (Rorty 1991b). It may be that 'two groups are not talking about the same things if they talk about them very differently, if wildly different beliefs and desires are aroused in them by these things' (ibid.: 103).

Another writer, Michel Foucault, grapples with the Enlightenment, which he argues offers the promise of human emancipation yet has given rise to the domination of totalising views or discourses.

KNOWLEDGE, POWER, SURVEILLANCE AND THE BIRTH OF THE INDIVIDUAL

From *Madness and Civilisation* [1961] (1965) to *The History of Sexuality* [1976] (1986), Michel Foucault explores the historical contingency of knowledge; 'the epistemological space specific to a particular period' that establishes 'what ideas can appear, what sciences can be constituted . . . what rationalities can be formed, only, perhaps, to dissolve and vanish soon afterwards' (Bellour 1966; cited in Miller 1993: 150). Foucault offers the postmodern claim of contingency a series of historical accounts of how 'regimes of truth' arise from, and give rise to, knowledges and rationalities, how contingent entities come to be constituted. Madness, the body and humanity itself, he argues, have no intrinsic nature outside the forms of sensibility of their periods. Each system of thought, of understanding, gives rise to classifications, whether of madness, disease or of the body. These classifications create their own subjects that are subjected to penetrating and scrutinising gaze.

We can take two strands from Foucault's writing to apply to the issues raised in this research. The first is the notion of systems of knowledge or discourses as ways in which power is gained, exercised and transmitted. The second is the place of surveillance as an integral technology of an increasingly 'disciplinary' society and an embodiment of the Enlightenment quest to dispel the areas of darkness in humanity and make all things knowable through the procedures of observation, recording, measurement; a particular form of rationality. We can understand and explore both Western society at large and the individual modern organisation using this image.

Knowledge and power

Foucault saw the 1960s as a period in which 'institutions, practices, discourses' became increasingly vulnerable to criticism. 'A certain fragility', he claims, 'has been discovered in the very bedrock of existence' (Foucault 1980b: 80). This criticism came from a variety of 'dispersed and discontinuous offensives', such as certain anti-psychiatric discourses. But against the activities of particular, local theorising, he sees the inhibiting effect of totalising theories – for example, those of Marxism, psychoanalysis or functionalist and systematising theory in general. Foucault argues that systematising theory masks or silences local knowledges so that they become subjugated and 'disqualified'. Such contingent knowledges have been set against and surrounded by 'the tyranny of globalising discourses' (ibid.: 83). His historical method, his 'genealogical' approach, has been to

> entertain the claims to attention of local, discontinuous, disqualified, illegitimate knowledges against the claims of a unitary body of theory which would filter, hierarchise and order them in the name of some true knowledge and some arbitrary idea of what constitutes a science and its objects.
>
> (ibid.: 83)

Science, or to be more precise, 'the effects of the centralising powers which are linked to the institution and functioning of an organised scientific discourse,' was, for Foucault, one such 'globalising discourse'. From a genealogical point of view, health policy and practice in Western societies can be seen as controlled by and extending the control of globalising discourses of science. Genealogies are 'anti-sciences' in that they expose the historical contingency of universal principles. He responds to the frequently asked question of whether Marxism (or psychoanalysis or semiology of literary texts) is, or is not, a science by asking

> about our aspirations to the kind of power that is presumed to accompany such a science. . . . What types of knowledge do you want to disqualify in the very instant of your demand: 'Is it a science?' . . . When I see you straining to establish the scientificity of Marxism, I do not really think that you are demonstrating once and for all that Marxism has a rational structure and that therefore its propositions are the outcome of verifiable procedures; for me you are doing something altogether different, you are investing Marxist discourses and those who uphold them with the effects of a power which the West since Medieval times has attributed to science and has reserved for those engaged in scientific discourse.
>
> (Foucault 1980b: 85)

However, the disinterment of these buried knowledges runs the risk of their re-colonisation:

> . . . those unitary discourses, which first disqualified and then ignored them . . . are, it seems, quite ready now to annex them and take them back into the fold of their own discourse . . . are we not in danger of ourselves constructing, with our own hands, that unitary discourse to which we are invited, perhaps to lure us into a trap.
>
> (ibid.: 83)

Foucault claims that the complex relations of power that permeate a society could not exist without the activity of 'discourses of truth'. 'We are subjected to the production of truth through power and we cannot exercise power except through the production of truth' (Foucault 1980b: 93). He argues that a discourse of kingly 'right' has, since the Middle Ages, masked, or effaced, the domination at its heart. Foucault's project has been to expose both the brutality and the latent nature of its practice, and investigate the multiple forms of subjugation found within society. This subjugation is found at its extremities, in specific institutions (for example health care organisations) and is investigated in its particular instances (at our particular point in political, economic and intellectual history). He explicitly turns away from a concern with intention and motivation, away from asking 'who then has power and what has he in mind?' to an examination of how things work at the level of ongoing subjugation, how subjects are progressively formed by all the mechanisms of subjection. Radically and in a much quoted and sometimes criticised passage (Hartsock 1990), Foucault refuses to understand power as a possession of particular groups:

> Power . . . is not that which makes a difference between those who exclusively possess it and retain it, and those who do not have it and submit to it. Power must be analysed as something which circulates, or rather as something which only functions in the form of a chain. It is never localised here or there, never in any body's hands, never appropriated as a commodity or piece of wealth. Power is employed and exercised through a net-like organisation. And not only do individuals circulate between its threads; they are always in the position of simultaneously undergoing and exercising this power. They are not only its inert or consenting target; they are always also the elements of its articulation. In other words, individuals are the vehicles of power, not its points of application.
>
> (Foucault 1980b: 98)

Far from crushing individuals, power actually has given rise to and constitutes the individuality which some have seen as the antithesis of power. I will argue that nurses in this study forged a subjectivity out of their experience of workplace exploitation. Foucault argues not for a 'descending' analysis of power – an analysis of how it is distributed – but an investigation of particular, specific manifestations of power, each with its own mechanisms and history. It is after this that the analyst must show how local techniques and technologies of power 'are invested and annexed by more global phenomena and the subtle fashion in which more general powers or economic interests are able to engage with those technologies' (Foucault 1980b: 99). (This is the approach of the present research.) An analysis that starts and finishes, for example, in terms of class domination lacks specificity. We need to investigate the processes of power and describe them in detail and then go on to show how they have become 'economically advantageous and politically useful . . . colonised and maintained by global mechanisms'. It is not the fact of exclusion from society of, for example, madness, that needs to be investigated but the mechanisms of that exclusion, for example the medicalisation of sexuality or madness.

Foucault offers a theory of society that we can attempt to bring to bear on the present study of organisations; a theory of countermovements, of the entrapping effect of two different discourses. In contemporary democratic society we hear a discourse and experience a legislation based on public right, the social body and each citizen's delegative status. This has come to function in a way that conceals the actual procedures of a second, closely linked discourse of disciplinary coercion 'whose purpose is in fact to assure the cohesion of this same social body' (Foucault 1980b: 106). Disciplines engender their own discourses, not, today, discourses of kingly sovereignty and right but of normalisation. The first step in the creation of such a disciplinary society is the formation of apparatuses of surveillance.

Surveillance

In *Discipline and Punish* (Foucault 1977), Foucault documents the transformation during the seventeenth and eighteenth centuries of the exercise of power and control over populations. Spectacular exhibitions of kingly sovereignty and terror characteristic of seventeenth-century Europe had turned, one hundred years later, into the efficiency of meticulous observation effected by continuous visibility or its ever present possibility. I will argue that the organisations under study in this book can be understood as exemplars of the disciplinary institution. The highly visible torture of the single transgressor is replaced by a silent and invisible gaze directed at the many. The development of the idea of a social contract can be seen as a step between these two. Through such a contract 'the right to punish has been shifted from the vengeance of the sovereign to the defence of society' (ibid.: 90). The offender, like the intransigent surgeon or irrational nurse, has become the common enemy.

Military training was one manifestation of a new focus on the body as an object to be analysed, manipulated and trained to infinitesimal degree:

> The human body was entering a machinery of power that explores it, breaks it down and rearranges it. A 'political anatomy', which was also a 'mechanics of power', was being born; it defined how one may have a hold over others' bodies, not only so that they may do as one wishes, but so that they may operate as one wishes, with the techniques, the speed and the efficiency that one determines.
>
> (ibid.: 138)

The practices of enclosure, whether of the military compound, the school, the hospital or the factory, along with such surveillance, create what Foucault terms 'disciplinary space', which involves a science of partitioning individuals in an optimal way to facilitate 'knowing, mastering and using' them. (Foucault 1977: 143) By assigning each individual its place, the supervision of the individual and the simultaneous work of all are made possible. Such partitioning, whether achieved through architectural, conceptual or temporal means – through the timetable – reflected the eighteenth-century interest in the problem of classifying the myriad diversity of things, zoological, economic or bodily. Classification brought order and mastery. The regulation of time became more important and, in certain circumstances, more closely linked to the maximisation of profit: 'How can one capitalise the time of individuals, accumulate it in each of them, in their bodies, in their forces or abilities, in a way that is susceptible of use and control? How can one organise profitable durations?' (ibid.: 157).

In the sense that 'strict training' creates from a confused multitude of bodies, well-ordered individuals, 'discipline "makes" individuals' (Foucault 1977: 170).

One major mechanism for effecting such discipline was the technology of hierarchical observation. The art of ever more penetrating seeing became a characteristic of the seventeenth and eighteenth centuries. Our attention has

been attracted to the metaphors of light and seeing associated with the
Enlightenment project of human understanding; Richard Rorty speaks of
Western notions of knowledge as dominated by 'Greek ocular metaphors'
(Rorty 1980: 11) and Derrida of Cartesian images of 'natural light' as the light
that makes manifest the truth (Derrida 1982b: 267). Managers in this study
made much use of visual metaphors for understanding. Foucault speaks about
'observatories' of human activity:

> Side by side with the major technology of the telescope, the lens and the
> light beam, which were an integral part of the new physics and cosmology,
> there were the minor techniques of multiple and intersecting observations,
> of eyes that must see without being seen; using techniques of subjection,
> and methods of exploitation, an obscure art of light and the visible was
> secretly preparing a new knowledge of man.
>
> (Foucault 1977: 171)

The military camp and the school building became exemplary 'observatories'
of the human body whose key characteristic was that

> a single gaze [should] see everything constantly. . . . A central point would
> be both the source of light illuminating everything, and a locus of conver-
> gence for everything that must be known: a perfect eye that nothing would
> escape and a centre towards which all gazes would be turned.
>
> (Foucault 1977: 173)

The effect of surveillance would not have been possible without a realisation
of the power of the realm of ideas. The Idéologues claimed that power over the
body can best be effected through the realm of ideas. '[T]he "pain" at the heart
of punishment is not the actual sensation of "pain", but the idea of "pain"'
(Foucault 1977: 94). Foucault quotes eighteenth-century criminologist, Servan
who suggested that the ideas of crime and punishment must be strongly linked
and:

> follow one another without interruption. . . . When you have thus formed
> the chain of ideas in the heads of your citizens, you will then be able to
> pride yourselves on guiding them and being their masters. A stupid despot
> may constrain his slaves with iron chains; but a true politician binds them
> even more strongly by the chain of their own ideas . . . on the soft fibres of
> the brain is founded the unshakeable base of the soundest of Empires.
>
> (Servan 1767: 35; cited in Foucault 1977: 102–3)

Systems of hierarchised, continuous and functional surveillance were extended
during the eighteenth century as such mechanisms brought with them hitherto
unexploited technologies of power. The spectacles of power that were enjoyed
one hundred years before, gave way to the anonymous and silent networks of

surveillance which traversed whole institutions and societies and in which the supervisors themselves were perpetually supervised. Foucault argues that hierarchised surveillance joined with a practice of 'normalising judgements' to form a technique central to modern society, that of the examination. Examination establishes over individuals a 'visibility through which one differentiates them and judges them' (Foucault 1977: 184). 'The superimposition of the power relations and knowledge relations assumes in the examination all its visible brilliance' (ibid.: 185).

The hospital came to be organised as an 'examining apparatus'. Inspecting visits from physicians became much more regular, in-depth and highly time-tabled. This altered the internal hierarchy of these institutions, with the result that their religious staff became relegated to particular roles. This is the age, argues Foucault, of the birth not only of *la clinique* – clinical medicine – but of the 'nurse'. The hospital, once little more than a poorhouse, became transformed into a site of knowledge, with the 'well-disciplined hospital' reflecting the new 'discipline' of medicine. Disciplinary power imposed on its subjects a principle of compulsory visibility: 'It is the fact of being constantly seen, of being able always to be seen that maintains the disciplined individual in his subjection' (Foucault 1977: 187).

The examination became the practice that held individuals in a mechanism of objectification, where power became manifested only by its gaze. The documentation associated with this practice introduced a previously unknown fascination with individuality, the writing of a whole archive of 'bodies and days'. The writing that accompanied the examination enabled the constitution of the individual as a describable, analysable object, constantly available to the gaze of a fixed body of knowledge. The individual became 'captured and fixed' in a mass of documentation. It also made possible a system of comparisons involving the measurement of overall phenomena and the variation between groups and the distribution of individuals within a 'population'. Thus towards the end of the eighteenth century, Foucault notes the entry of the individual as opposed to the species into the emergent clinical sciences. The individual became 'a case' whose individuality was brought across the threshold of describability by the techniques of disciplinary surveillance, what Foucault terms the 'turning of real lives into writing' (Foucault 1977: 192). In that it emerged from this disciplinary practice, the individual became an effect and an object both of knowledge and of power.

> We must cease once and for all to describe the effects of power in negative terms: it 'excludes', it 'represses', it 'censors', it 'abstracts', it 'masks', it 'conceals'. In fact power produces; it produces reality; it produces domains of objects and rituals of truth. The individual and the knowledge that may be gained of him belong to this production.
>
> (ibid.: 194)

Individuality was a 'positive product' of disciplinary surveillance.

One architectural 'discovery' facilitated at once constant surveillance and individualisation. This was the so-called 'Panopticon'. Its champion was Jeremy Bentham (1748–1832). Bentham's Panopticon, with its architecture whether of a prison or hospital ward enabling total visibility of its subjects, stood out for Foucault as the emblem of 'subjection by illumination'. 'It was just what [doctors, penologists, industrialists and educators] had been looking for. [Bentham] invented a technology of power designed to solve the problems of surveillance' (Foucault 1980a: 148). The Panopticon was an emblem of a disciplinary age:

> . . . at the periphery, an annular building; at the centre, a tower; this tower is pierced with wide windows that open onto the inner side of the ring; the peripheric building is divided into cells, each of which extends the whole width of the building; they have two windows, one on the inside, corresponding to the windows of the tower; the other, on the outside, allows the light to cross the cell from one end to the other. All that is needed, then, is to place a supervisor in a central tower and to shut up in each cell a madman, a patient, a condemned man, a worker or a schoolboy. By the effect of backlighting, one can observe from the tower, standing out against the light, the small captive shadows in the cells of the periphery . . . each actor is alone, perfectly individualised and constantly visible.
>
> (Foucault 1977: 200)

Its ultimate effect was that: 'An inspecting gaze, a gaze which each individual under its weight will end by interiorising to the point that he is his own overseer, each individual exercising this surveillance over, and against, himself' (Foucault 1980a: 155).

As with the panoptic hospital ward advocated and described in detail by Nightingale (1883), the arrangement enables the chief inspector to watch over subordinates as well as inmates and for the inspector to be watched over by a superior. There are striking comparisons with the modern organisation under central control:

> The Panopticon may even provide an apparatus for supervising its own mechanisms. In this central tower, the director may spy on all the employees that he has under his orders: nurses, doctors, foremen, teachers, warders; he will be able to judge them continuously, alter their behaviour, impose upon them the methods he thinks best; and it will even be possible to observe the director himself. An inspector arriving unexpectedly at the centre of the Panopticon will be able to judge at a glance, without anything being concealed from him, how the entire establishment is functioning.
>
> (Foucault 1977: 204)

Since the seventeenth and eighteenth centuries, the electronic, over and above the optical, has lowered unimaginably further the 'threshold of describability'.

The quest is still for ever clearer visibility. Many nurses in the present study appeared poised on the brink of interiorising this gaze through regular self-recording of the details of their activities.

If Foucault's work examines the historical processes that have masked the operation of power in society, it is possible to examine textual practices in a similar way. Deconstruction argues that texts characteristically efface the method of their operation, their construction of and reliance upon dualism, the way in which their central organising principles are displaced to some point outside the text as a 'first principle'.

DECONSTRUCTION, METAPHOR AND INTENTION

Deconstruction began as a response to structuralism and is sometimes referred to as post-structuralist criticism. The project of European structuralists was to discover underlying laws or structures behind and beneath the whole range of human sign-making. Semiology, or the study of such signs, was proposed as a scientific basis for such a quest. (See Chapter 3 for a fuller explanation.) Anthropologist Claude Lévi-Strauss, for example, suggested that all myths may be aspects of a single great myth being produced by the collective mind of humanity. Like the other writers discussed earlier, Jacques Derrida was sceptical of the search for universal laws governing human sign-making. He argued that the search for such a unity amounted to a new version of an ancient quest for the lost ideal, 'whether that ideal be Plato's bright realm of the Idea or the Paradise of Genesis or Rousseau's unspoilt Nature' (Peterson 1992: 363). The structuralist search for 'centres of meaning' within texts, for him, derived from the logocentric belief that there is, somewhere, a reading of a text that accords with a 'God's-eye' reading. There are clear echoes here of postmodernism's critique of the Enlightenment pursuit of context free knowledge.

Deconstruction explores and exploits the discovery that a single text can be used to support seemingly irreconcilable positions. In offering an explanation or account of any text, one primary meaning for a work, the reader or critic necessarily (and perhaps conveniently) overlooks certain passages. J. Hillis Miller, American literary theorist, has suggested 'Deconstruction is not a dismantling of the structure of a text, but a demonstration that it has already dismantled itself' (Miller 1976). It is this exploitation of countertexts, the deliberate subversion of the initial reading of a text, that informs my treatment of textual data produced within this research. Such subversions may involve an analysis of metaphor and its place in argument, an examination and overturning of a text's dualisms and a radical approach to the question of intention and context. (A full account of their use in action is given in Chapter 3.) Here, however, in presenting deconstruction and summarising some of the work of Jacques Derrida, I introduce the theoretical orientation guiding these approaches.

Dualism

Derrida argues that as Westerners, influenced and shaped by the traditions of our philosophies, starting with the Greeks, we tend to think and express thought in terms of dualisms such as presence/absence, speech/writing – something is masculine and therefore not feminine, the cause rather than the effect. Edward Said, though not a name one might associate with deconstruction, makes a similar point: 'No identity can ever exist by itself and without an array of opposites, negatives, oppositions: Greeks always require barbarians . . . ' (Said 1993: 60). According to Derrida, such dualisms tend to contain implicit or explicit hierarchies as one element of the dualism is privileged, according to the world view of Western cultural tradition. Both the managers and nurses involved in this research constructed such dualisms involving, for example, the rational and the irrational or human care and financial concern.

The hierarchical opposition between speech and writing which is of particular interest to Derrida will be discussed later. Involved in such a hierarchy is the privileging of presence, 'the belief that in some ideal beginning were creative *spoken* words, words such as "Let there be light," spoken by an ideal, *present* God' (Peterson 1992: 361; original emphasis). Within a logocentric tradition, these original and originary words can now only be represented in speech and writing that is unoriginal, unreliable, open to misinterpretation and 'parasitic' on the original utterance. Derrida's approach to such hierarchies is not simply to reverse them and so perpetuate the same oppositional mode of thought, but to 'erase the boundary' between such oppositions in a way that fundamentally questions the order and values upon which they are based:

> . . . an opposition of metaphysical concepts (for example, speech/writing, presence/absence, etc.) is never the face-to-face of two terms, but a hierarchy and an order of subordination. Deconstruction cannot limit itself or proceed immediately to a neutralisation: it must, by means of a double gesture, a double science, a double writing, practice an *overturning* of the classical opposition *and* a general *displacement* of the system.
>
> (Derrida 1982a: 329; original emphasis)

Deconstruction works by demonstrating that the privileged element in a dualism, for example speech over writing, can equally plausibly be seen as secondary. For example, deconstruction can show how cause can become effect, and the marginal, central. The result is not a simple reversal of the old order but a more fundamental dislocation or displacement that undermines the metaphysical privilege given to the prior element. The 'literal and the figurative can exchange properties so that the prioritising between them is erased' (Peterson 1992: 365).

Metaphor at the root of metaphysics and metaphor in science

Derrida's uncovering of the activity of metaphor lurking within and behind that most abstract of sciences, philosophy, is a pattern for its disclosure in the purportedly rational argumentation of NHS managerialism.

In Derrida's approach to Socrates and Plato, in which he examines the role of metaphor within the argumentation of metaphysicians (Derrida 1982b), the distinction between the disciplines of philosophy and literary criticism is seen to dissolve. In his treatment of Aristotle and, in another essay, of linguistic philosopher John Austin (Derrida 1982a), he works to uncover the text working against the grain of the text's argument. Even the question he poses at the outset of *White Mythology: Metaphor in the Text of Philosophy*, becomes fractured, inverted and endlessly reflective:

> Is there metaphor in the text of philosophy? . . . Our certainty soon vanishes: metaphor seems to involve the usage of philosophical language in its entirety, nothing less than the usage of so-called natural language *in* philosophical discourse, that is, the usage of natural language *as* philosophical language.
>
> (Derrida 1982b: 209; original emphasis)

Derrida argues, as Nietzsche had done before him (Nietzsche 1994), that language is radically metaphorical in character. The metaphorical basis of philosophy, he argues, had been disguised and forgotten since the Socratic dialectic style of debate had monopolised all claims to reason and truth. For Socrates' student, Plato, the rhetorician-philosophers known as the sophists came to stand for 'verbal ingenuity mixed with persuasive guile' and were depicted as easily defeated by Socratic logic (Norris 1991: 60). Nietzsche, and later Derrida, argue that, in spite of his claims, Socrates was himself a 'wily rhetorician' and that:

> Behind all the big guns of reason and morality is a fundamental will to persuade which craftily disguises its workings by imputing them always to the adversary camp. Truth is simply the honorific title assumed by an argument which has got the upper hand . . .
>
> (ibid.: 61)

Furthermore, Derrida argues that metaphysics can only be spoken of metaphorically and metaphysicians, in their attempts to express abstract ideas, are constrained to live 'perpetually in allegory', with the faint imprint of the ancient fables appealed to by pre-Socratic Greek philosophers, still detectable in their most abstract of writings. '[T]hey dim the colours of the ancient fables, and are themselves but gatherers of fables. They produce anaemic [or white] mythology' (Derrida 1982b: 213). This approach enables Derrida to undermine the universalist claim of Western philosophy and its claim to have purged reason and logic of the deceptions of rhetoric:

> Metaphysics – the white mythology which reassembles and reflects the culture of the West: the white man takes his own mythology . . . for the universal form of that he must still wish to call Reason . . . metaphysics has erased within itself the fabulous scene that has produced it.
>
> (ibid.)

Searching for a metaphysical truth about metaphor inevitably leads us to metaphor; metaphor is like a coin, standing in for something else. Thought continually 'stumbles upon metaphor' (Derrida 1982b: 233). Making metaphor belongs to the *mimesis* (imitation) and language-making considered by Aristotle in his *Rhetoric* as the characteristic of humankind. Yet if it is proper and appropriate to humankind, it is a means to knowledge that is, for Aristotle, a subordinate one. Derrida paraphrases him: ' . . . it is not as serious as philosophy itself . . . metaphor, when well trained, must work in the service of truth, but the master is not to content himself with this, and must prefer the discourse of full truth to metaphor' (ibid.: 238).

If Aristotle and other Greeks considered metaphor ancillary to philosophy, closer to the present, Derrida draws our attention to historian Bachelard, who argues in a similar fashion when writing about metaphor in science. For Bachelard, 'metaphors seduce reason' (Bachelard 1938; cited in Derrida 1982b: 259) and tend to take over thought with their own autonomous life and imagery. Derrida notes, however, that in the field of the natural sciences, animistic or cultural metaphor may be so appropriate that 'one might be so tempted *to take the metaphor for the concept*'. Drawing on the work of Georges Canguilhem, Derrida examines the development of cellular theory, 'over which', according to Canguilhem, 'hover, more or less closely, affective and social values of co-operation and association' (Canguilhem 1969: 49). Biologist Hooke when first having observed the cell through a microscope, named it thus under the influence of an image of the honeycomb. But also, asks Canguilhem, 'who knows whether, in consciously borrowing from the beehive the term cell in order to designate the element of the living organism, the human mind has not also borrowed from the hive, almost unconsciously, the notion of the co-operative work of which the honeycomb is the product?' (ibid.: 48–49).

In short, metaphor cannot be consigned to the margins either of philosophy, of science or of language itself. Metaphor can be used to prize apart the layers of argument upon which is based the tyranny of totality and rationality.

Presence/absence and the question of intention

A consideration of intention as the final authority regarding the meaning of a text is vital to my treatment of the interviews and comments in this book. To begin this consideration, we must see how Derrida approaches the theories of Austin, for whom intention was a central concern.

In *Signature Event Context*, Derrida critiques Austin's speech act theory (see Chapter 3 for more detail about the work of John Austin) and explores in the process theories of meaning and traditional distinctions between speech and writing, which he finds untenable. He argues that within the Western tradition of what he calls 'logocentrism', since Plato, with its 'metaphysical longing for origin and ideals', speech has been privileged and writing has been seen as a kind of corrupt activity, parasitic upon speech. According to this philosophical tradition, speech and writing are successive but transparent stages in the representation of 'thought' and 'ideas' whose various structures do not influence the content of those original thoughts. However, the invention of writing, while enabling people to make their thoughts known to 'absent persons' (Derrida 1982a: 312) gave rise to its dangerous yet inevitable 'drifting' in meaning, its separation from the present consciousness of its originator as the final authority of this meaning. Derrida places Austin within this tradition of thinking because of his attempt to anchor the meaning of an utterance in the conscious intention of its speaker so that different types of speech act (for example, those utterances he termed performatives), such as the giving of promises, can be classified on the basis of intention. Derrida argues that the absence of the addressee and, indeed, of the addressor in writing is in need of more critical examination:

> For the written to be the written, it must continue to 'act' and be legible even if what is called the author of the writing no longer answers for what he has written, for what he seems to have signed, whether he is provisionally absent, or if he is dead, or if in general he does not support, with his absolutely current and present intention or attention, the plenitude of his meaning, of that very thing which seems to be written 'in his name'.
>
> (ibid.: 316)

Part of the *very structure* of the written word is that it is separable from the present and the context of its inscription, and is citable in new contexts. However, having said this, Derrida also claims that even speech is subject to similar 'drifts' in meaning through the possibility of its placing in different contexts:

> Every sign, linguistic or nonlinguistic, spoken or written . . . as a small or large unity, can be *cited*, put between quotation marks; thereby it can break with every given context, and engender infinitely new contexts in an absolutely nonsaturable fashion. This does not suppose that the mark is valid outside its context, but on the contrary that there are only contexts without any centre of absolute anchoring. This citationality, duplication, or duplicity, this iterability of the mark is not an accident or an anomaly, but is that . . . without which a mark could no longer even have a so-called

'normal' functioning. What would a mark be that one could not cite? And whose origin could not be lost on the way?

(Derrida 1982a: 320–321; original emphasis)

'Meaning is context-bound, but context is boundless' summarises Culler (1983: 123). But what of intention? Intention cannot be considered as a single fixed point of origin:

When questioned about the implications of an utterance I may quite routinely include in my intention implications that had never previously occurred to me. My intention is the sum of further explanations I might give when questioned on any point and is thus less an origin than a product, less a delimited content than an open set of discursive possibilities . . . intentions do not . . . suffice to determine meaning; context must be mobilised.

(ibid.: 127–128)

In other words, an utterance acts in different ways depending on the context in which it is placed. Intentional, original and metaphysically privileged meaning, if such a thing exists, cannot set a boundary around all future or possible meanings. How then can we understand the task of the reader of literature, historical documents, the transcripts of interviews with NHS managers or the status of any human utterance or mark? Deconstruction offers the suggestion of an aporia, or impasse, a double movement between two opposed yet simultaneous approaches:

If we say that the meaning of a work is the reader's response, we nevertheless show, in our descriptions of response, that interpretation is an attempt to discover meaning in the text. If we propose some other decisive determinant of meaning, we discover that the factors deemed crucial are subject to interpretation in the same way as the text itself and thus defer the meaning they determine.

(Culler 1983: 132–133)

Finally, and crucially for this research, deconstructive literary critics reject the traditional distinction between the literary text and the critical work which comments upon that text (de Man 1979). For them, the poetic or literary work has no sacrosanct and unique autonomy. Conversely, they also deny the notion that the work of criticism has a privileged status over and above the works it comments upon. The critical enterprise itself is bound to use the same persuasive techniques as the texts it attempts to unravel. In the same way, this research claims no privileged access to truth about the texts it analyses and attempts to deconstruct. This work is ultimately rhetorical, as is the case, I would argue, for any inquiry that, unlike this one, claims access to a metaphysical grounding, whether that grounding be located in scientific methodology or in the privilege of direct experience or insight. The status I would wish to claim for it is neither more nor less than a cultural production alongside the novel or the prophecy.

Summarising

So do these deconstructions explain texts, show what they mean? Derrida would argue that anyone seeking a single, correct meaning to a text is imprisoned by a structure of thought that would oppose two readings and consider one as correct and right, and not incorrect or wrong. Deconstruction argues that literature defies the laws of Western logic, laws of opposition and non-contradiction. Texts don't say 'A and not B'; they say 'A and not A' (Peterson 1992). To the reader who finds my readings of managers and nurses later in this book implausible, improper or perverse, I reply that the text is not a bearer of stable meanings. Unlike some qualitative researchers, I do not consider my task as being to faith-fully seek the truth in texts, to represent the origins of their intention, somehow directly, to the reader. I think of it rather as to place these texts in new, perhaps uncomfortable, contexts, to wrest their meaning out of the hands of those groups who lay claim to their ownership.

Literature will always evade any theory we attempt to encompass it with. J. Hillis Miller asserts that this does not make way for a critical free-for-all. He maintains that it is possible to present a reading which is demonstrably wrong (Miller 1976; cited in Peterson 1992: 375). What he argues is that critics are mistaken in any assumption that the meaning of a text is going to be single, unified and logically coherent. The best readings give the best account of the heterogeneity of a text. 'It is the very incompatibility of discourses within literary texts that makes literature mysterious, problematic, worthy of attention' (Peterson 1992: 362).

When we go on to consider the post-structuralist maxim, 'there is nothing outside of the text' (Derrida 1976: 158), in other words, a world understood by us and given meaning by us can be considered textual, we may be tempted to replace Peterson's 'literature' with 'NHS research'. This chapter has presented the arguments of postmodern writers who have questioned the truth claims of science, philosophy and certain approaches to textuality. It has also summarised the work of those who have made the relationship between knowledge and power explicit. The next chapter explores disruptions between fields of inquiry and goes on to explain more carefully some details of the analysis of discourse and deconstruction as they apply to this project.

3 Erasing the boundaries: speech into text, comment into text

Two erasures can be performed which open up a space within which certain redescriptions can be offered. The first is the freeing of words from the context of research data – interview transcripts, written survey data, field notes – into a context of text; the freeing of words from the context of authorial intention, of manifestations of a thinking, knowing, self-expressing subject (Foucault 1972: 55) into objects of inquiry in themselves with meanings that escape any notion of individual intention. In a sense, these texts create their own speaking and writing subjects.

The second erasure is of the boundaries between long-standing, yet, in a sense, arbitrary fields and styles of inquiry; between sociology and philosophy or between literary theory and policy studies. A novel space is available in which these disciplines can be drawn upon with the aim of making the familiar problematic.

THE BLURRING OF LITERARY CRITICISM AND OTHER DISCIPLINES

Since the 1980s, there has been an expansion in critical explorations that have straddled the boundaries between disciplines such as sociology, anthropology and philosophy. Literary theory, psychoanalysis and biblical studies have also been drawn into this new space. In some ways, the precursor to this tendency was structuralism which, in the middle decades of the twentieth century, called together endeavours aimed at detecting underlying structures, particularly linguistic structures, beneath the phenomena that were traditionally studied by workers in a range of fields (Bell 1985). More recently, this quest for commonality gave way to a sense that such knowledge was impossible to arrive at. Nevertheless a focus on structures and on language remains.

Perhaps another strand is to be found in what has become known as critical theory. According to Kincheloe and McLaren, critical theory, 70 years after its development in Frankfurt in Germany, still manages to 'disrupt and challenge the status quo'. Its approach is characterised by a belief that 'all thought is fundamentally mediated by power relations' (Kincheloe and McLaren 1994:

138–139) and by an emancipatory aspiration. Inquirers who espouse this approach can be found working in the fields of literature, law and a whole range of social and cultural studies.

This move has involved a distinct disrespect for existing demarcations. Jacques Derrida, philosopher and literary theorist, critiques Freud (Derrida 1978). Harold Bloom, another literary theorist offers biblical exegesis (Bloom 1987); so does feminist philosopher Hélène Cixous (1993). Philosopher Richard Rorty writes in depth about literature and anthropology (Rorty 1991b) while Michel Foucault offers detailed art criticism (Foucault 1970; 1983). A landmark collection of essays exploring the dialogue between feminism and postmodernism includes writers with backgrounds in philosophy, communication studies, modern language and political science, offering critiques of these subjects as well as of issues more traditionally the terrain of psychologists, psychotherapists and sociologists (Nicholson 1990), while a blend of semiology, sociology, ethnography and management studies has recently emerged as the movement known as organisational symbolism (Turner 1990). In 1993, Edward Said, writing about how cultural productions have been implicated in imperialism, prefaces a quotation from poet T. S. Eliot in this way: 'although the occasion as well as the intention of his essay is almost purely aesthetic, one can use his formulations to inform other realms of experience' (Said 1993: 1). Later he comments: 'The tendency for fields and specialisations to subdivide and proliferate . . . is contrary to an understanding of the whole, when the character, interpretations, and direction or tendency of cultural experience are at issue' (ibid.: 13)

Jocalyn Lawler, in her examination of 'somology', a study of the body, comments that the body in its totality has fallen between the discourses of academic disciplines, disciplines that themselves to a large extent reflect the lives of Western white males (Lawler 1991).

Literary theorist Jonathon Culler, writing in the early 1980s, detected the emergence of a field of inquiry within an as yet unnamed domain. It could not be labelled 'literary theory' because many of its works did not address literature explicitly. It could not be called 'philosophy' either because it included attention to De Saussure, Marx, Freud, Goffman and Jacques Lacan as well as Hegel and Nietzsche. 'It might be called "textual theory"', ventured Culler, 'if *text* is understood as "whatever is articulated by language"' (Culler 1983: 8; original emphasis). Works from this genre act as 'redescriptions that challenge disciplinary boundaries'. Richard Rorty sensed that in England and America, literary criticism had taken the place accorded to philosophy, 'as a source for youth's self-description of its own difference from the past' (Rorty 1980: 168).

At such a time, the autonomous existence of disciplines is challenged. Christopher Norris sees Derrida as undermining the privileged status accorded to philosophy as sovereign dispenser of reason (Norris 1991). Derrida achieves this, Norris argues, by critically examining metaphorical and other figurative devices at work in the texts of philosophy. Doing this, he challenges the notion that reason can somehow transcend language and arrive at 'a pure, self-authenticating truth or method' (ibid.: 19). Norris goes on to write:

In this sense Derrida's writings seem more akin to literary criticism than philosophy. They rest on the assumption that modes of rhetorical analysis, hitherto applied mainly to literary texts, are in fact indispensable for reading *any* kind of discourse, philosophy included.

(ibid.; original emphasis)

Culler explores a little further this deconstruction of the hierarchy between 'serious' philosophical texts and 'nonserious' literature. However, a whole range of discourses: sociology, health legislation, research reports can be grouped with the 'serious':

The notion of literature or literary discourse is involved in several of the hierarchical oppositions on which deconstruction has focused: serious/ nonserious, literal/metaphorical, truth/fiction . . . philosophers, to develop a theory of speech acts, construct a notion of 'ordinary language' and 'ordinary circumstances' by setting aside as parasitic exceptions all non-serious utterances, of which literature is the paradigm case. Relegating problems of fictionality, rhetoricity and nonseriousness to a marginal and dependent realm – a realm in which language can be as free, playful and irresponsible as it likes – philosophy produces a purified language which it can hope to describe by rules that literature would disrupt if it had not been set aside. The notion of literature has thus been essential to the project of establishing serious, referential, verifiable discourse as the norm of language.

(Culler 1983: 181)

Foucault finds parallels between literary and scientific text when he draws attention to the complex relationship between a statement, its author and the subjects that the statement creates (Foucault 1972). The relationship between an enunciating subject (created by a text) and the author is not one of simple correspondence. He rejects the view that this ambiguity is peculiar to, and characteristic of, literature. A mathematical text, for example, may evoke at various points, a number of different subjects, making statements of different kinds, adopting different stances towards the text. These kinds of shift of subject that are understood implicitly by the reader as they read, become an area of scrutiny for Foucault. The point is that Foucault would subject 'books, texts, accounts, registers, acts, buildings, institutions, laws, techniques . . . ' to the same approach (ibid.: 7).

In contrast, others have observed similarities between the activities of those engaged in the pursuits characteristic of different disciplines, but without questioning the different epistemological status usually accorded the two. For example, Strong observes similarities between the activities of the sociologist and the writer of fiction but he still leaves unquestioned, in a way that Derrida does not, a certain privilege granted to science. For Strong, science is, or at its best can be, 'disinterested', a commenter, showing a 'unique rigour', 'a collegial pursuit of independent truth' in which 'ideological, practical and aesthetic aims

. . . constantly threaten the distinction between' sociology and fiction (Strong 1983: 71–73). Atkinson also looks at the blurred boundary between the telling of 'fact' and 'fiction'. He examines the persuasiveness of the ethnographic account and the often unconscious use ethnographers have made of literary devices in 'their constructions of reality' (Atkinson 1990).

SPEECH ETC. INTO TEXTS

A brief history of a 'turn to language'

The influence of structuralism and post-structuralism has, since the 1960s and 1970s, led workers within a range of disciplines including philosophy, sociology and psychology to place a concern with language at the forefront of their inquiry. Part of this reorientation has been the realisation that language is structured in a way that reflects and constantly adds stability to existing power relations. Dale Spender (1980), looking at women and Edward Said (1978; 1993), writing about nations colonised by Western powers have argued that such groups have not only their identity but also the structure of existence defined for them by powerful outside groups. Colonisation, writes Said, gives rise to 'structures of feeling' created by the coloniser for the colonised (Said 1993: 9) so that there is an 'inability to conceive of any alternative' (ibid.: 14). Part of this defining is achieved through the structures of language made available that systematically silence and estrange marginalised groups and leave them with few alternative ways to live in and describe a world that becomes ever more alien to them. 'There is no use looking for other, non-imperialist alternatives; the system simply eliminated them and made them unthinkable' (ibid.: 26).

One manifestation of the 'turn to language' is discourse analysis.

Discourse analysis

A broad range of theoretical perspectives underpin activities that go under the name of discourse analysis (Potter and Wetherell 1987), from measurement-orientated analysis of the structures of a text (Renkema 1993), through analysis of conversation and turn-taking (Sacks *et al.* 1974) to more broadly ideological studies (Thompson 1984). In the health care setting notable work has been done by Silverman (1997) and Atkinson (1995). Discourse analysts vary in the amount of confidence with which they claim the workings of cause and effect in the operation of texts and it is probably fair to say that the field is factional. To avoid confusion, it is vital to make clear what kind of discourse analysis I will *not* be developing in this book. I am not creating an analysis of the structure of conversation, with its turn-taking and other sequences, nor with producing 'models' of argumentation or numerical accounts of the reading process. These approaches, I suggest, do not do justice to the inevitable ambiguity of texts. It will become clear that what I am concerned with is the link between knowledge, language, power and identity made manifest by analysis of the philosophical positions implicit in and drawn upon by the talk of managers and nurses. Discourse analysis can help investigate how speakers make a particular construction appear natural.

Potter and Wetherell (1987) locate the foundations of this range of activities in the speech act theory of British philosopher John Austin (1962), the discipline of ethnomethodology, semiology, the structuralist 'science of signs' proposed by Ferdinand De Saussure (1974) and developed by Roland Barthes in order to stimulate social criticism (Barthes 1972; 1985), and the rise of post-structuralism associated with the writings of Michel Foucault, Jacques Derrida, Jean-François Lyotard as well as Barthes.

Austin's contribution lies in his perspective on speech which constituted, in 1955, a radically new departure in the philosophy of language. He deflected attention away from the truth or falsity of statements, the discovery of which had exercised the logical positivists. Through his theory of speech acts he asks us first to consider whether some types of utterance are principally important for what they *do* rather than for how they describe things. He called such written or spoken utterances *performatives* while descriptive utterances were termed *constantives*. Later, Austin went on to overturn this distinction: '*all* utterances state things *and* do things' (Potter and Wetherell 1987: 17; original emphasis). In other words utterances have force as well as meaning. Language is a tool to get things done. Ethnomethodologists such as Garfinkel (1967) use a similar approach in studies of how 'ordinary people' make sense of life and achieve and maintain 'membership' of particular groups; for example nurse or manager. Ethnomethodology is the study of the 'taken-for-granted' assumptions which give structure and meaning to everyday life. Often these taken-for-granted assumptions are embedded in the features of conversation. Although broadly concerned with how social life is put together, these studies explore, in social settings, the 'reflexive' nature of talk, in other words how language does not just describe actions or situations but, in part, constitutes or formulates these actions and situations. Ethnomethodologists look at what speakers are *doing* with their talk by studying how speech and other face-to-face behaviour constitutes reality 'within actual mundane situations' (Maynard 1989).

The third, and perhaps the most significant, theoretical tradition out of which discourse analysis has grown is semiology, or, more broadly speaking, structuralism. Swiss linguist Ferdinand De Saussure (1857–1913) explored the distinction between any particular concept such as a dog, which he termed the *signified*, and the speech sound associated with it, the *signifier*. The combination of both are termed the *sign*. His central principle concerns the arbitrary connection between signifier and signified. Not only are the speech sounds associated with certain concepts arbitrary – they vary from language to language – but the concepts themselves are indeterminate. Again, using examples from various languages, De Saussure demonstrates that certain distinctions and categories are available to speakers of some languages but not to the speakers of others. 'The world can be conceptually partitioned in endless different ways' (Potter and Wetherell 1987: 25). Barthes even suggests that language brings both power and servility, its categories compelling us to say certain things (Barthes 1996). What gives meaning to a sign is not some intrinsic quality it possesses but its place within a particular system, its difference from other signs. It is this idea that lies behind his notion of a science of the signs used within societies. In this science, 'signs' would include not only language, but any realm to which meaning has been applied, such as fashion or architecture.

Barthes developed the notion of signification to include 'second level signification', or myth, where a sign can become signifier to a new signified. For example, Barthes writes about a travel guide – the *Blue Guide* – '[t]he picturesque is found any time the ground is uneven' (Barthes 1972: 74). The *Guide*'s 'overstress[ing] of hilliness', according to Barthes, is linked to a nineteenth-century Protestant morality which combined the cult of nature with Puritanism, 'regeneration through clean air, moral ideas at the sight of mountain-tops, summit climbing as civic virtue, etc.' '"*The road becomes very picturesque (tunnels)*"' he quotes, and comments, 'it matters little that one no longer sees anything, since the tunnel here has become a sufficient sign of the mountain' (ibid.).

In the present study both 'manager' and 'nurse' might be understood as having mythic qualities; the manager standing for effectiveness, organisation, power, the nurse for selflessness, healing and compassion. Paradoxically, both stand for areas of hope for humanity, but within starkly different systems of thought. In Chapters 6 to 8 we can see how these two groups drew upon negative mythic notions of each other to help establish and maintain their own identities.

Discourse analysis can be considered a structuralist pursuit if we understand structuralism as 'an investigation of a text's relation to particular structures and processes . . . [in which] . . . [l]anguages and structures, rather than authorial self or consciousness, become the major source of explanation' (Culler 1983: 21), or post-structuralist if we consider the following distinction: 'Structuralists are convinced that systematic knowledge is possible; post-structuralists claim to know only the impossibility of this knowledge' (ibid.: 22). I would like to suggest that post-structuralist writers, such as those named, have avoided the idealised and static approaches of semiologists and speech act theorists and offered more dynamic and radical analyses of text, language and discourse.

Discourse analysis has been located by some within the 'critical post-modernism' sketched out by Kincheloe and McLaren (1994), a frame of reference that combines critical theory's concern for political action resulting in emancipation with postmodernism's philosophical suspicion and focus on text. For example, Lupton discusses some of the characteristics of 'critical discourse analysis' in the light of post-structuralist thinking (Lupton 1995). These feature, in particular, a fluid sense of the subjectivity of the speaker. I discuss some of the possible contradictions inherent in the proposition of 'critical postmodernism' in Chapter 9.

What is a discourse?

> Discourses do not simply describe the social world, they categorise it, they bring phenomena into sight. . . . once an object has been elaborated in a discourse, it is difficult *not* to refer to it as if it were real. Discourses provide frameworks for debating the value of one way of talking about reality over other ways.
>
> (Parker 1992: 4–5; original emphasis)

Parker offers seven criteria for distinguishing discourses: a discourse is realised in texts, it is about objects, it contains subjects, it is a coherent system of meanings, it refers to other discourses, it reflects on its own way of speaking, and is historically located. In addition a discourse often supports institutions, reproduces power relationships and has ideological effects (ibid.).

Put another way, we could suggest that our interpretation is freed from the primacy of the subjectivity of the speaker and becomes an investigation of the structures of a text and 'how it gives birth to a world' (Ricoeur 1996: 152).

Where are discourses found? In texts. Where and what are texts? If we search for discourses in texts, we can find texts virtually everywhere:

> I want to open up the field of meaning to which discourse analysis could be applied beyond spoken interaction and written forms by saying that we find discourses at work in *texts*. Texts are delimited tissues of meaning reproduced in *any* form that can be given an interpretative gloss.
>
> (Parker 1992: 6; original emphasis)

In an interview, Derrida argues against the accusation that deconstruction is a form of 'textualism' which transforms everything 'real' into a book:

> Now you well know there is nothing to this, that the concept of text, once re-elaborated, leaves nothing outside itself, and is especially irreducible to the book or to writing. It does not exclude the referent or the real or history: quite the reverse, if one could say so. . . . I recall this briefly to underline the fact that we do not speak merely of writings 'small' or 'great', canonical or otherwise, but of historico-political places, if you will, within which these writings are inscribed and exceeded.
>
> (Derrida 1992: 200)

What is meant by objects and subjects?

'The reference to something, the simple use of a noun, comes to give that object a reality' (Parker 1992: 8). De Saussure argued that 'The object is not given in advance of the viewpoint: far from it. Rather one might say that it is the viewpoint adopted which creates the object' (De Saussure 1996). For Foucault, discourses are 'practices that systematically form the objects of which they speak'

(Foucault 1972: 49). Foucault's work has looked, for example, at the constitution of sexuality as such an object (Foucault 1984a). Objects within this research include 'dead wood', people in an organisation who are depicted by others as failing to achieve their potential (see Chapter 7), or a 'patient/client', a kind of person, devised by health professionals, who has a certain relationship with professional care givers.

There is a particular kind of object – the subject. The subject either 'speaks, writes, hears or reads the texts discourses inhabit':

> A discourse makes available a space for particular types of self to step in. It addresses us in a particular way. When we discourse analyse a text, we need to ask in what ways, as Althusser (1971) put it when he was talking about the appeal of ideology, the discourse is hailing us, shouting 'hey you there' and making us listen as a certain type of person.
>
> (Parker 1992: 9)

For example, a discourse on 'dead wood' positions us, or invites us to listen as responsible, tax-paying, organisational members committed to effectiveness. A discourse about 'patient/clients' inclines us to respond as compassionate, human individuals. Not only this, but the person or institution giving expression to a discourse can place themselves in a range of available subject positions including the two above. However, this subject need not be a consistent one; it can change during the course of a discourse and can even appear to inhabit a number of spaces simultaneously. I will show some notable instances of this sometimes uncomfortable multiple positioning later in this chapter.

Discourse analysis challenges the Enlightenment's supposition of a unitary, autonomous self and focuses attention instead on how the self is talked about and on the 'grammatical and metaphorical self' (Potter and Wetherell 1987: 106–107). Post-structuralism has provided the realisation that psychological models of the self are historically and culturally contingent. In fact, Foucault has suggested that it is the discourse that constitutes the subject rather than the converse. For him there is no individual unified subject lying at the origin of a discourse (Foucault 1972). The political relevance of such an awareness is that the self may be articulated in a discourse aimed at maximising the chance of its version of events being taken seriously. This may have significant consequences for the positioning of people in society. In other words, some articulations of the human subject establish and maintain patterns of domination and subordination.

HOW CAN WE APPROACH THESE TEXTS?
DECONSTRUCTING THE AUTHOR AND HIS/HER
INTENTION

So far we have seen that there is a precedent for approaching the whole range of cultural production as texts, that is, places where discourses may be situated and analysed. An analysis of a text can benefit from detailed attention to the effects of language. Yet it might still be asked how far research 'data' can be approached in the same way as literary texts. Surely the considered lines of the poet are entirely different stuff to the nurses' hurried comments written on the last inches of a questionnaire or to the spontaneous, hesitant or politically astute words of a health service manager captured by the tape recorder? What justifies approaching them in a similar manner? Three points of similarity can be drawn.

First, as I will go on to argue, and hopefully demonstrate, in this chapter, language, through allusion, metaphor and other rhetorical devices always contributes to the effect of a text and can reinforce, or undermine, broader discursive moves. Second, drawing from post-structuralist literary theory, we can question the privilege usually given to the conscious intention of the speaker in analysis of a text. I discussed this in Chapter 2 in the section on deconstruction and offer a further explanation below. Third, as we shall see, in a brief exploration of the work of Derrida over the following pages, there is always some aspect of a text *working against itself.*

Rhetorical effects support discourse

In the comments and transcripts of this research, no less than in literary production, language is doing more than acting as the unremarkable, neutral and fleeting building blocks out of which rational meaning is built. It is also doing another kind of work which it may accomplish through a range of rhetorical devices such as rhythm, alliteration, through more complex allusion, or by metaphorical means. The analysis of discourse as described by Parker, and Potter and Wetherell acknowledges the role played by language but perhaps emphasises broad interpretative processes, rather than close attention to such rhetorical effects. However, as Culler says of deconstruction, 'when [analysis] concentrates on the metaphors in a text or other apparently marginal features, they are clues to what is truly important' (Culler 1983: 146).

Intentionality and text against itself

The issue of intentionality is debated both within literary theory and within the study of discourse in such a way that there is little useful distinction left between the two types of text. Parker suggests that the analysis of texts goes beyond the realm of conscious, individual intention into explorations of connotation, allusion and implication (Parker 1992 : 7). He also wishes, however, to preserve a sense that there may be an 'author' behind a text as 'source and arbiter of a true meaning'. This point is strongly disputed. Some literary theorists have seen criticism as essentially an elucidation of an author's purposes. A proponent of the New Criticism of the 1940s and 1950s, Cleanth Brooks, based his critical approach on the principle that 'the poet knows precisely what he is doing' (Brooks 1947; cited in Culler 1983: 218). However, more recently others, like

Barthes, have argued that the location of authentic meaning lies within the reader:

> [T]he text is not a line of words releasing a single 'theological' meaning (the 'message' of an Author-God) but a multi-dimensional space in which a variety of writings, none of them original, blend and clash . . . [however] . . . there is one place where this multiplicity is focused and that place is the reader, not, as was hitherto said, the author. . . . a text's unity lies not in its origin but in its destination.
>
> (Barthes 1977: 146, 148)

It is between these two poles that the iterative, unresolvable account of reading proposed by post-structuralism lies.

Eagleton summarises some of the debate over literary intention and the extent to which it is fixed, discoverable or even existent:

> What is the meaning of a literary text? How relevant to this meaning is the author's intention? Can we hope to understand works which are culturally and historically alien to us? Is 'objective' understanding possible, or is all understanding relative to our own historical situation? There is . . . a good deal more at stake in these issues than 'literary interpretation' alone.
>
> (Eagleton 1983: 66)

Eagleton rejects the idea that meaning is something prelinguistic that an author (or speaker) wills, which is then 'fixed' in the form of material signs. Literary works, and the same can be said, I would argue, of the texts of the interviews in this research, are not the 'private property' of the speaker for the very reason that they are the products of a language that is social before it is personal. As De Saussure suggested, the categories and practices of thought reflect the structures of language available to any speaker. It is discourse as textual practice rather than as a clue to thoughts, themes or preoccupations (Foucault 1972: 138) that will be of interest in this study. In later chapters, I will refer to the notion of language having its own independent life, 'speaking through' the positions of various subjects (Chapter 6) or of certain discourses being so 'available' to the nurses and managers involved in this research that they almost cannot help but adopt them, particularly under the pressure of having to defend positions they feel are under threat (Chapter 7).

This attention to metaphor is linked to deconstruction's habit of overturning hierarchies, metaphysical oppositions and dualisms:

> to deconstruct a discourse is to show how it undermines the philosophy it asserts, or the hierarchical oppositions on which it relies, by identifying in the text the rhetorical operations that produce the supposed ground of the argument, the key concept or premise.
>
> (Culler 1983: 86)

The result of this approach to texts is not an elucidation of their unifying concept or meaning but the production of a 'double, aporetic logic' (ibid.: 109), an impasse, an account of the words of managers and nursing's leaders, for example, that offers a counterinterpretation to their widely accepted, 'authentic' meaning. What emerges from this aporia is a loss of privilege for what was considered basic, foundational, authentic or pure. When Derrida considers intentionality as exceeded by the text, I take him to mean that the text's own explicit declarations can be subverted by the text itself. His detailed examination of Aristotle's writing on metaphor and philosophy (Derrida 1982b: 207–271) discussed in the previous chapter could be considered to achieve such an end.

To summarise, a close attention to the effects of language, or textual accomplishment, can support analysis and reveal in detail how certain discursive accomplishments are achieved. To this end, I will adopt a number of approaches to the text. Owing much to deconstructive literature, they include an examination of:

- metaphor and rhetorical effects;
- dualism;
- multiple subject positions;
- the 'parasitic' – how certain instances of a phenomenon are 'accounted for' or set aside as being marginal and dependent upon mainstream instances.

In addition to these approaches that focus closely on the text, two broader strategies should be outlined. The first reflects Culler's summary of deconstructive activity:

> (A) one demonstrates that the opposition [set up by a text] is a metaphysical and ideological imposition by (1) bringing out its presuppositions and its role in the system of metaphysical values – a task which may require extensive analysis of a number of texts – and (2) showing how it is undone in the texts that enunciate and rely on it. But (B) one simultaneously maintains the opposition by (1) employing it in one's argument (the characterisations of [various oppositions] are not errors to be repudiated but essential resources for the argument) and (2) reinstating it with a reversal that gives it a different status and impact.
>
> (Culler 1983: 150)

Secondly, we can pose three questions when examining the diversity of statement that can be found within a discourse:

> (a) . . . who is speaking? Who, among the totality of speaking individuals, is accorded the right to use this sort of language? Who is qualified to do so? Who derives from it his own special quality, his prestige, and from whom, in return, does he receive if not the assurance, at least the presumption that what he says is true?
>
> (Foucault 1972: 50–52)

For example, who derives their prestige and authority from and who has claimed ownership of terms such as 'financial accountability', 'strategic planning', 'professional preciousness' or from terms such as 'intuition', 'expert' or 'professional care'?

> (b) We must also describe the institutional *sites* from which the doctor [speaker] makes his discourse, and from which this discourse derives its legitimate source and point of application.
>
> (ibid.; original emphasis)

Foucault considers the hospital, private practice, the laboratory and the (medical) library as sites from which the discourse of modern medicine has developed, each site constituting its own particular type of authority. Possible sites for managers in this research might be the boardroom, the document – trust application, business plan, annual report or, for the nurse, the site is close to the patient.

> (c) The positions of the subject are also defined by the situation that it is possible for him to occupy in relation to the various domains or groups of objects . . .
>
> (ibid.)

Foucault sees the doctor occupying a number of positions: the observer, the questioner or the listener and argues that technology allows the doctor to change the perspective that he is able to take. In the present research it is above all the computer that enables or promises to enable the manager to scrutinise the activity of his or her staff and so to speak as observer; it is human resources expertise that enables him or her to speak as one who has access to 'what makes the worker tick' and financial accounting procedures that enable him or her to speak as responsible actor in the public interest.

In the rest of this chapter I offer some examples of the approaches to textual analysis that I outlined above.

SOME EXAMPLES OF ANALYSIS

Rhetorical effects

The following is a comment added to a job satisfaction questionnaire. It adopts a range of rhetoric to support its argument that nursing is in danger of being wrested away from what the writer sees as its traditional orientation toward human values:

> I'm dissatisfied with 'simple is best' attitude in nursing being replaced by 'Let's complicate, high tech' attitude coming in. Empathy, bedside manner, care. These words are being replaced by customer, computer, audit, budget.

Why don't we start looking down at our hands with our thoughtful eyes and using common sense and intelligence use those hands practically, to care for our patients.

(staff nurse in community hospital)

Although this comment makes much use of dualism, I would like to concentrate on its use of metaphor and other specific rhetorical effects. The first part of the comment sets the context for the second, more unresolvable movement. The comment is introduced by the word 'dissatisfied', carried over, perhaps ironically, from the response format of the numerical part of the questionnaire. Taken out of the context of one of a range of purportedly emotionally neutral responses, here it regains its character as a blunt and direct adjective. The first two sentences set the scene, telling of the intrusion into nursing of a contrasting and alien set of values, a barrage of characteristics that sound pedantic and insensitive when listed one after the other, 'customer, computer, audit, budget'. While not intrinsically undesirable, the way this commenter lists them, along with their alliteration, 'customer, computer', makes us experience them as such, particularly when contrasted with strongly human, comfortingly traditional terms, 'empathy, bedside manner, care'. The term 'replace' is an understated, rather abstract verb that suggests quiet, perhaps chilling rationality. Also, her use of the passive mood, 'being replaced by' rather than 'are replacing' enacts a passivity and powerlessness that the speaker perhaps feels within her profession. This enables or encourages us, the readers, to see nursing as the victim in this situation. Nursing is having something done to it. '[C]oming in' suggests at once something of a fashion or fad identifying this business orientation as superficial but also suggests an intrusion or penetration, both with suggestions of inappropriateness or violence. These effects work together having an accumulative persuasive effect on the reader.

The third sentence is unusually figurative. Appropriately, for a discourse about personal care delivery, its metaphor is one of the body. It can be understood in a number of ways but a possible reading is as a plea for a body (nursing, or perhaps the Trust) that is at the moment divided against itself to become integrated, for eye and hand to work together in a way that figures a combining of 'intelligence' and 'common sense'. (A well-known biblical passage, Paul's first letter to the Corinthians (1 Cor. 12: 15) uses the same image of disagreement between the parts of the body as an image of a disunited organisation.) In a common approach to the body (Walsh and Middleton 1984: ch. 7), its upper organs are associated with rationality, 'thoughtful eyes'. In this case, however, it is the lower organs, hands, which are given a privilege. They are associated with the physical world of practical action 'caring for our patients' which is at once the end (purpose) of nursing and of the statement. That this can be understood as a statement calling for balance and integration is surprising from its context because the first part of the statement strongly emphasises the values of simplicity and direct practicality. One way of reading this is to see it as a desire to reconnect and reground the rational, nonphysical aspects of an organisation, profession or society that are becoming dominant and disconnected from physical, practical concerns. However, the vigour with which the 'new attitude' is rejected makes such a resolution problematic.

In summary, we can see that the details of language can be linked to broad political issues and give an insight into the subject position being adopted by the speaker/writer.

Dualism

In the present study, nurses describe how they see management as having different priorities and values to themselves. A great many comments erect a series of 'us–them' dualisms. This is done by collecting together a range of attributes or concepts and contrasting them with another range, either explicitly or implicitly. This dualism becomes the given, unquestioned ground for arguments about values and moral themes. Looking at one such dualism, caring (with which nurses identified) is given a moral privilege while financial concerns, associated with management, are characterised as morally suspect. From within this system, irony and punning can be drawn upon with relative ease to enact and reinforce the moral posture of the commenters.

> What price can we put on care?
>
> (nursing auxiliary)

> Money seems to be the thing [senior management] want to CARE about most of all.
>
> (nurse manager; original emphasis)

However, we could suggest that the moral purity of the caring ethos is infected by financial consideration; it is offered by some nurses as the basis of the entitlement of their patients and clients to nursing services (national insurance contributions)

> [I] . . . give the patients I visit the care they are entitled to . . .
>
> (clinical nurse specialist)

and it is also involved in the establishment and maintenance of the nurses' expertise and credibility, their authority to care, in the form of occupational training and continuing membership of a professional group. The rhetorical question asked by the first speaker thus can be answered in specific terms. In one sense, a price can be put on caring. The clear distinction between the components of the opposition is blurred and the hierarchy loses its power.

Multiple subject positions

Possible contradictions within a discourse are a source of interest for the analyst. In the present study such contradictions can be located even within the utterances of individuals. The following speaker, a nurse in an 'upper-middle' management position, like many whose words have contributed to this research, makes contradictory utterances within even the same sentence. Speaking about the possible impact of the NHS reforms on her staff she said:

> 'There has been a sort of deliberate policy that we shouldn't get people worried before they had to be worried.'
>
> (community manager)

A meaning can only be forced out of this passage by examining the tension between a number of logical contradictions: a policy that is at once a 'policy', a 'deliberate policy' and a 'sort of deliberate policy' and a reference to the management of information that carries contradictory suggestions of both caring and concealment. In another passage from the same interview there is a similar contradiction:

> 'I mean its a big responsibility with the numbers of staff that we've got and people dependent on *their* professions [i.e. their livelihoods] and not only [?this] first and foremost, always, comes our patients and clients of our service, but next, very closely after that comes our staff and that actually is an even greater responsibility lying on my shoulders.'
>
> (ibid.; original emphasis)

This short section of the interview transcript was sent to the manager who uttered it for permission to include it in a report. The manager asked for the passage not to be included as it stood because it included a suggestion that her priority was her staff's welfare rather than the welfare of the clients they served. 'If I did say that, I didn't mean it' was her explanation. It could be argued that this manager is attempting to occupy two subject positions simultaneously, one as an individual (a nurse) who cares for and feels a high degree of responsibility for her staff during a period of extreme uncertainty, the other as a manager who is working at a time when the rhetoric of consumer led service has priority. She appears to feel that to even be suspected of expressing any other priority (i.e. that her staff's welfare could be more important) would be considered politically unacceptable in her organisation. Her 'impossible' language in which patients and staff are *both* her top priority, reflects the 'impossible' situation she appears in and forces her to adopt a number of subject positions simultaneously.

Parasites

As we have seen, part of a deconstructive task has been close analysis of a text's structures of argument, particularly its reliance on metaphor and hierarchy. The maintenance or imposition of hierarchy often depends on the treatment of the special case. For example, in a text (or a culture) where speech is privileged above writing, writing is set to one side as a particular instance of speech, an impure and corrupt exception that relies for its existence and its definition upon speech in such a way that an opposition emerges. In this sense writing can be constructed as parasitic upon speech. A deconstructive reading of such an argument would involve demonstrating, possibly by using only the resources available in the original argument, that the opposite conclusion (in this case that speech is a particular case of writing) is equally, if not more, tenable. In the present study it could be argued that the norms and consensus appealed to by many managers are achieved by acts of exclusion. This echoes Rorty's observation that objectivity or rationality has been generally conceived of in terms of the level of 'general agreement among sane and rational men' (Rorty 1980: 337). 'In other words, objectivity is constituted by excluding the views of those who do not count as sane and rational men: women, children, poets, prophets, madmen' (Culler 1983: 153). In the present study managers could exclude or treat as a special case the views of, at least sections of, their nursing staff on the grounds that 'they trained at a time when the world was a very different place' (local services manager) or that they belong to a fearful and insecure profession (chief executive), or were suffering from a 'mega-neurosis about skill-mix' (chief executive), or that they believed senior management was 'Machiavellian' with a 'hidden agenda', or were 'worried' by new language (nurse executive) or belonged to the '5 per cent' of staff who represented an 'intractable problem' (nurse executive) or were 'threatened by management concepts' (chief executive). For all of these reasons, the views of a great many nurses could be made marginal to a mainstream objectivity which, by contrast, characterised itself as modern, rational, confident, open, founded on consensus, flexible and corporate.

An alternative reading of some of these statements can overturn this dualism and reveal staff as realistic, perceptive and 'canny' and management as operating from an irrational system of beliefs. According to many managers, staff believed, without good cause, that skill-mix changes would involve cost-cutting and a reduction in the quality of service. At the time of the study, evidence was accumulating to support the fact that skill-mix adjustments were widely considered by managers as methods of cost reduction (Buchan and Ball 1991) and also arguments that quality of care could be compromised by such measures (Audit Commission 1991; Car-Hill *et al.* 1992). Indeed, suspicion that managers had a particular agenda for cost containment could not be considered far-fetched in the light of the managers' own aim of maximising capital return and reducing unit costs. Finally, regarding the supposed irrationality of the nursing workforce one manager suggests that he and staff have a different relationship to language:

'I think people are worried by language like that – "a competitive edge", "competing in the market place" and "customers". We've never talked

of any of that stuff before. I actually think we are more efficient an organisation because we've addressed those kinds of issues.'

(nurse executive)

He appears to be claiming that the 'new' language like that he quotes, gives rise
to irrational fear for many nurses while for the organisation, the talking of such
notions into existence is a channel for rationality and efficiency. However, it
could be argued that the same phrases that alert staff to changing times stand
as icons for those committed to the ideologies of competition and operational
efficiency and that managers stand in exactly the same nonrational relationship
to such language. This is precisely the operation of discourse.

I have given some examples of the ways that texts can be approached that offer
alternatives to either simple summarising or the search for 'authentic' intention.
They are approaches with origins in deconstruction, first associated with literary
criticism and theory, and in the analysis of discourse, the foundations of which
can be located in speech act theory and semiology, structuralism and post-
structuralism. These approaches show how the always contingent structures
of language can lend authority to certain ways of talking while disqualifying
others. They highlight the struggles for power that are enacted in a rhetorical
battleground.

The nurses who commented in this research drew strongly on discourses of
moral activity but before we look at these texts and the texts of managers, we
need to look at some of professional nursing's 'official' discourses because they
provide a background and contrasting context in which to place the comments
of the nurses.

4 Locating nursing within the discourses of the Enlightenment*

For more than three decades, it has been my theoretical posture that caring is the essence of nursing and the explanadum for health and well-being. It is also the explanadum for the survival of human cultures and civilisations.

(Leininger 1990: 19)

Simplifying to the extreme, I define *postmodern* as incredulity toward meta-narratives.

(Lyotard 1979: xxiv; original emphasis)

INTRODUCTION

The issues of power and knowledge are central to nursing. As a predominantly female occupation existing in a patriarchal society and working in close association with a medical profession which has successfully maintained a formidable power base, it would be astonishing if it were otherwise. Nurses have generally been more comfortable understanding themselves as working on a project of liberation from oppression than acknowledging themselves as implicated in the very same power moves as those who they see as oppressing them. Many nurses are able to critique effectively the medical institution as engaged in a process of maintaining a significant power base, marshalling biomedical knowledge as one of its resources, but they appear to often take at face value the nursing profession's own rhetoric of holism, patient advocacy, professionalism or feminism, unwilling to understand those arguments and rhetorics as cultural resources, discourses that are adopted to further the profession's desire for power. The sincerity of the great majority of those in nursing who have taken up these arguments does not mean that these discourses do not function as 'technologies of power'. Indeed, there is no reason to assume that the champions of biomedicine or managerialism are themselves empty of idealism, radicalism, or passionate, even naive, belief.

---

* The title of this chapter, though not its content or argument, is taken from a paper delivered with enviable aesthetic style by Kim Walker at The Adventure of Nursing Practice through Research Conference held at the University of Sydney, Australia, June 1994.

This chapter explores some of the 'official' nursing discourses adopted by nursing's leaders from the days of Florence Nightingale to the 1990s. Contingent upon the times and cultures in which they were voiced, they reflect the dominant or at least promising-looking language and values of their day. As will be seen, there are notable differences between the discourses of nursing's leaders and those nurses involved in this research.

Even apart from this difference, which is easy to stage, it has been difficult to do justice to the complexity and contradiction of the various projects nursing leaders have engaged in, the discursive spaces they have been drawn into as they have sought to represent the identity and the value of the nurse. They have been drawn to spirituality, theory, technicism and science, to conventional and more radical notions of professionalism, to the politics of liberation, to managerialism and economic utility, to New Right politics, to postmodernism. It will come as little surprise that I can find no ground from which to make final evaluative judgements between these that do not simply, and perhaps unwittingly, set up camp within any one of these spaces or upon some other ground. However, in tracing some of these discursive strategies, I can at least point to some of the unintended, constraining consequences of some of these positions, how they disparage and disqualify other positions or how they re-enact a discourse that they appear to be rejecting. It is also possible to speculate on the genealogy of some of these positions.

I argue that many of the profession's leaders have searched for epistemologies that maximise nursing's professional and cultural standing – a difficult task as, after quasi-religious beginnings, nursing had to steer between the Scylla of biomedicine and the Charybdis of 'caring as women's work'. As we shall see in this chapter, at times the rhetoric of nursing leaders claims radical departure from Enlightenment and scientific paradigms but their arguments sometimes produce the same quest for a defining power over others or for power through association with the language games of powerful groups.

NURSING'S HISTORY

Histories of nursing have been told and retold. Nowadays Florence Nightingale is as likely to be heaped with blame as revered. Although she has been described as responsible for the 'early feminist roots' of nursing (Chinn and Wheeler 1985), her reputed emphasis on tasks and procedures is blamed for the slow emergence of a knowledge base for nursing (Jolley and Allan 1991). Early nursing's failure to separate 'autonomy from altruism', according to Reverby, has resulted in nurses accepting a duty to care but without contributing to how that care was constituted (Reverby 1987). Nightingale's characterisation of nursing, and nurse training, as character development, a calling with strict adherence to orders passed through a female hierarchy, has been seen to lead to an unempowering posture and to the reinforcement of the notion of a separate sphere of activities for women: 'Nursing was built on a model that relied on the concept of duty to provide its basis for authority' (ibid.: 7). Such a collective attitude has been seen to 'legitimise men's right to supervise and superintend the behaviour of women' (Rafferty 1993a: 51).

Nurses' moral performance seems to have been subject to intense scrutiny, not just from men. The principal of efficient surveillance lies at the heart not only of Bentham's Panopticon but of Nightingale's ward design. She argues that poor ward design contributed to lack of hospital discipline. In Nightingale's *Notes on Hospitals* (1883) discussed by Baly (1986: 5), she records meticulous details of a ward layout which allows not only the penetration of the maximum of fresh air and light but also enables nurses to be under constant supervision. And even as early as 1865 she had suggested in a letter to H. Bonham Carter that nurses' meals ideally should be eaten in the ward scullery or attended by the superintendent. 'The whole establishment must be so constructed that the probationers' dining rooms, day rooms, dormitories and the matron's residence and office must be put together and the probationers under the matron's immediate hourly direct inspection and control' (Nightingale 1865; cited in Baly 1986: 5). In fact Sir Joshua Webb, architect of the new model prisons advised on the structure of the nurses' home in Liverpool (Baly 1986).

Ann-Marie Rafferty describes how in the last 40 years of the nineteenth century the emphasis in the character and objectives of nurse training shifted from the moral to the professional. The new nursing elite looked to medicine for its inspiration in developing a model of professional organisation (Rafferty 1993a). Although new nurses, she argues, were influenced by the women's movement and by expanding employment opportunities for women, 'assuming the mantle of medicine meant . . . identifying closer with medical interests, values and practices' (ibid: 55). Pro-registrationist Mrs Bedford Fenwick wanted nursing to be legally recognised as a distinct profession with a central controlling body of its own but Nightingale thought that registration by the state would interfere with the 'conventual discipline' possible within hospitals. Opponents of registration rejected claims for similarity, and by implication, intellectual and social parity with medicine. They argued that the medical emphasis was scientific and intellectual while 'by contrast, nursing was qualitatively different and "good" nursing could not be tested by examination' (Rathbone 1892; Rafferty 1993a: 56). Similar claims for an unquantifiability about nursing are sometimes raised today, though since the days of contracting, the 'internal market' and 'clinical effectiveness' such a discourse has become less legitimate and voiced less openly.

Nursing registration was discussed in a context where women's suffrage was high on the country's political agenda. 'The nurse question is the woman question', said Mrs Bedford Fenwick (Rafferty 1993: 195). Nursing reformers saw their profession's struggle to be differentiated from, and stand alongside, the male bastion of medicine as part of women's wider struggle for equality. However, as Rafferty argues, groups keen to secure certain privileges may adopt the same traditions advocated by those perceived as already having achieved success (Rafferty 1992). She gives examples of how the organisation of nursing history began to mirror that of medicine, for example in its appeal to exemplary figureheads and foundational principles. Nutting and Dock (1907), early historians of nursing, attempted to construct an illustrious history by appealing to the legitimacy of science to argue for the supreme status of 'caring'. According to Russian zoologist Kropotkin, whose work they drew upon, Darwin was mistaken; it was in caring and co-operation, rather than combat and competition, that the key to evolutionary success lay. Using this approach, they attempted to form an association between a supposedly universal – even the supremely important – characteristic and the professional activity of a particular group. More modern versions of this kind of move will be discussed later.

Today's legacy

The view of nursing as an essentially moral activity has been seen as giving rise to a heritage of anti-intellectualism, leaving nursing today as 'a field of practice without a scientific heritage . . . a profession without the theoretical base it seems to require' (Johnson 1974: 373). From this point of view, the development of nursing theory can be seen as a duplication of a characteristic approach of the medical profession and itself becomes a means of professionalisation (Jolley and Allan 1991). However, Rafferty argues that the application of a medical form of organisation to further the autonomy of nurses has created a legacy from which contemporary nurses have arguably yet to break free. The 1980s 'new nursing' with its stress upon individualism and the personal characteristics of the nurse (Salvage 1985) echoes the moral emphasis of an earlier period (Rafferty 1992), and some have argued that it also accorded well with the New Right thinking characteristic of the period (Masterson 1996).

Chandler appears perhaps more questioning than many nurses when writing about professionalisation (Chandler 1991). She argues that the greater and more apparent the theoretical and abstract pool of knowledge claimed by a group, the greater the social status accorded to them. She sees the United Kingdom Central Council for Nursing, Midwifery and Health Visiting (UKCC) Project 2000, in which nurse training moved into higher education, and which I will discuss later, in terms of a strategy for professional advancement. She notes, however, that others, such as Jane Salvage, characterised it more as a survival strategy (Salvage 1988). For Chandler, the wish of some nurses to move away from a biomedical foundation is problematic. This move runs the risk of reinstating the principle of nursing and caring as women's work. The strategy of many nurses, therefore, has been to make their closest alliances with other theoretical disciplines, the social and behavioural sciences and in this way still maintain theoretical and academic credentials. Chandler senses, however, like philosopher Richard Rorty, that the epistemologies associated with these disciplines are still considered 'softer' and as having less status than those of biomedicine (Rorty 1991c). However, critiques of scientific development by Kuhn (1970) and Capra (1983) have become foundational texts for those, like the theoreticians of nursing, whose work I will examine soon, who wish to move away from restrictive notions of inquiry and truth while retaining equally valid claims to truth.

NURSING THEORIES AND MODELS

In the 1980s, a number of American nursing academics published reflections on the profession's theoretical enterprises of the previous decades. By that time an array of theories and conceptual models of nursing practice were available for examination, comparison and evaluation, and there was a concern to clarify the intellectual origins of this theorising. I will not attempt to catalogue the models and theories here. Rather my purpose is to explore the character of their presentation in the context of modernity. I will look first at two major, but in many ways contrasting, American reflections from the 1980s and then at one further contribution from the UK, from the early 1990s.

My central argument is that these writers place the possibility of autonomous professional practice upon a newly elaborated and scientifically derived theoretical foundation and describe this as a coming of age of the profession. I would argue that this move parallels modernity's accounts of its own advance, for example Kant's telling of the history of humanity in his essay *Was ist Aufklärung?* (What is Enlightenment) (1784), with both its celebration of a newly acclaimed human reason, and its promise and challenge of emancipation from traditional authority (Foucault 1984b). The development of nursing theories is placed explicitly within the context of Kant's account of human understanding by one writer. The narratives woven by Fawcett (1984) and Meleis (1985) about the efforts of nurse theorists over the past decades appear strongly influenced by evolutionary theory and at points approach triumphalism. They relegate, I would argue, certain groups within nursing to the role of hindrance to its proper fulfilment and they present the ascendancy of their own aims as the 'development' of the profession.

They describe the 1960s and 1970s as a period characterised by elaboration of nursing theories and models. The impetus for such an enterprise was the desire to forge a range of 'concepts' that were distinct from those employed within medicine and to disentangle them from those of other disciplines. This change in nursing is presented as a 'journey' with 'stages' and 'milestones' (Meleis 1985: 7), as a development, an advance, an 'evolution of nursing' and its champions are lauded as 'pioneering' (Fawcett 1984: viii). The establishment in 1955 of the journal *Nursing Research* is described as nursing's first significant 'milestone' after Florence Nightingale, offering 'confirmation that nursing is indeed a scientific discipline and that its progress will depend on whether or not nurses pursue truth through an avenue that respectable disciplines pursue, namely research' (Meleis 1985: 13). Indeed, the era of theory building is seen as the culmination of nursing's history. It can even be understood as a Platonic return to an original but lost realm in the shape of Nightingale's environmental model, forgotten since the days of the domination of illness-orientated medicine.

Regarding science, these documents are ambiguous as perhaps is nursing's history itself. The authors of these accounts offer critiques of the 'positivistic' science of 'reductionism, quantifiability, objectivity and operationalisation'

(Watson 1981) and suggest that nurses have been hampered in their theorising by paying allegiance to these notions. They argue that nursing practice, in contrast, has been more 'open, more variable, relativistic and subject to experience and personal interpretations' (Meleis 1985: 74). Nursing knowledge became the battleground upon which adherents of these views fought for influence. However, in spite of this, the authors appear to have little reservation about claiming the status and disciplinary benefits ascribed to the authority of science. Indeed, science is presented as the new, or rediscovered, foundation for nursing.

The benefits of developing conceptual models of nursing are all too clear; 'The thinking of Karl Marx, Albert Einstein and Sigmund Freud is paramount in the shaping of the 20th century world. Each had a conceptual model' (Lippitt 1973; cited in Fawcett 1984: 230). The close links between the 'scientific' ability to 'predict consequences', and professional autonomy and power are clearly spelled out:

> The autonomy of a profession rests more firmly on the uniqueness of its knowledge, knowledge gathered ever so slowly through the questioning of scientific inquiry. Nursing defined by power does not necessarily beget knowledge. But knowledge most often results in the ascription of power and is accompanied by autonomy.
>
> (Fuller 1978: 701)

Additionally, in focusing such power, conceptual models offer a disciplinary potential because they can bring unity to the myriad 'private images' held by nurses (Fawcett 1984). Theorising and model building, therefore, can be a means of turning power inwards and exercising control over nurses themselves. Both Fawcett and Meleis acknowledge the presence of different groups within nursing who hold conflicting interests. Some of these groups were either actively sceptical of theoretical activity or were uncommitted to the profession and its projects. Although Meleis is able to present nursing's theoretical enterprise as one that enhances the professional and academic standing of women, certain women are excluded; 'non-career-orientated individuals, those who were looking for an occupation that allowed them to get in and out conveniently as their families demanded' (Meleis 1985: 37). Commitment to a 'professional career' is equated with 'scholarly productivity' and the theoretical realm:

> women in general, have been conditioned to consider a professional career as secondary to family and home. It is a situation that has not allowed the energies of women to be released for more creative endeavours such as theory development and theory testing.
>
> (ibid.: 41)

These women, then, are excluded from the theoretical and pioneering realms in Meleis' history of nursing's achievement. Her own group of nursing career academics appears to be privileged in the role it played and in its access to the power that can flow from the theoretical enterprise. This is a further aspect of modernity, that certain groups can claim access to reason and its manifestations and present reason and rationality as the basis for their own interested position.

Considering these models from the perspective of UK nursing in the 1990s, Kitson suggests that they 'explain what nurses do' (Kitson 1993). Her catalogue of nursing theories is introduced by a problematic encounter with medicine, in the form of a doctor's wife, also a nurse, who voices, with a gaucherie worthy of farce, one of nursing's deep fears:

> 'I don't believe in all of that nonsense. I'm just an ordinary nurse. Anyway you don't need a lot of brains to be a good nurse. It's just basic care and common sense. I don't know why all these nurses want to go to university . . . why didn't they do medicine in the first place?'
>
> (ibid.: 26)

Kitson's discursive project is to beat what she describes as the 'task duty-doctor's assistant' model into a 'patient-centred ethically driven collegiate activity'. She cites the three categories of theory developed by Meleis: needs-based theories, interaction theories and outcome (or holistic) theories (Meleis 1985). Each looks to different fields of established theory for their development, for example interaction theories are said to draw upon Roger's psychotherapeutic theories and phenomenology. Three stages in what is termed the evolution of concepts of caring are then introduced. The first stage, caring as duty, is traced to Nightingale's desire to protect the vulnerable from 'unscrupulous women masquerading as nurses'. This is characterised as primitive and unhelpful: its moralistic and religious overtones do not square well with more intellectualised and professionalised conceptualisations. As well as this, it is said to have had a detrimental impact on nurses' emotional life as studies such as that by Menzies (1960) are said to demonstrate.

A discourse of caring as therapeutic relationship – the second phase – emerged in the 1970s and 1980s. Within this view, nurses develop more emotionally focused aptitudes such as empathy, respect, love, compassion and bring them to bear by practising techniques such as touching, instruction and other stress-alleviating measures. Proponents of this view include Leininger (1978) and Rogers (1980). The third and most recent form of discourse associated with caring is 'caring as an ethical position'. Watson's work sees the goal of caring as to help those cared for to 'a higher level of harmony in mind, body and soul' (Watson 1985) while Benner argues for nurses to care for patients 'as they see fit'. Benner seeks to move away from rules, bounding care towards the individual, autonomous judgements of practitioners in particular circumstances. The nurse's good decisions depend upon her ethical stance, which also equips her to perform caring functions. For Benner, caring is not altruism but rather an evolutionary stage in human development (Benner and Wrubel 1989). Kitson then superimposes these two frameworks to give rise to a table showing nine possibilities. The resulting range of possible positions seems to represent at once pragmatic ways of thinking, between which the practitioner can move, and intellectual and ethical developments. It is interesting to observe that the technology of the table, as Foucault has argued regarding its emergence in the nineteenth century, is used as a mechanism of representation and organisation (Foucault 1989), as well as of surveillance and control:

> These small techniques of notation, of registration, of constituting files, of arranging facts in columns and tables that are so familiar to us now, were of decisive importance in the epistemological 'thaw' of the sciences of the individual . . . one should look into these procedures of writing and registration, one should look into the mechanisms of examination, into the formation of the mechanisms of discipline, and of a new type of power over bodies.
>
> (Foucault 1977: 190–191)

Practitioners unfortunate enough to be caught in 'traditional' theories and values can, according to Kitson, be 'moved' through the matrix. The most valued intersection is that between the caring-as-ethical position and holistic nursing. The needs-based/caring-as-duty model is 'definitely passé', although it finds many echoes in the comments of nurses involved in this research. It is left very much open to question how such thoughts and conceptualisations 'influence the way we interact with our patients' as it is suggested they should.

While the models are discussed in terms of their differences, they share a common quest to locate the activity of nurses within an authoritative discourse, and, in turn, to exercise authority over those nurses by defining them in terms of these places on the table. Perhaps the 'inconsistencies' that are said by Kitson to trouble those nurses who have not clarified their conceptualisations represent such disqualified forms of knowledge spoken of by Foucault (1980b: 85).

NURSING AND RESEARCH

Goodman describes the early days of research in nursing and its emergence after the Second World War. The foundation of the first UK university nursing departments in the 1960s, and research units in the early 1970s, appear as milestones. The purpose that research was expected to serve is revealed by the key question: 'is nursing research generating and validating the knowledge necessary for clinical nursing practice?' (Goodman 1989: 100–101). It was intended to be scientific and, above all, applied. However, the promotion of nursing research and nursing education as a whole became central to nursing leaders' attempt to move the profession away from a stereotypical female image of 'intuition' and lack of question, an approach for which Nightingale has been credited. Macleod Clark and Hockey open their collection *Research for Nursing: A Guide for the Enquiring Nurse* with the metaphor of combat: 'Nurses must develop the ability to defend their decisions and actions on a scientific rather than intuitive or conventional basis. It is on this ability that their claim to professionalism rests' (Macleod Clark and Hockey 1981: 6).

Part of its quest for distinct identity involved the search for a research methodology that was appropriate to the issues as well as the values of nursing. Fawcett held that many nurses had been heavily, and unhelpfully, influenced by the philosophy of other disciplines (Fawcett 1983) while Leininger forcefully argued that would-be nurse researchers had been held in tyranny by the 'unassailable rightness' of quantitative approaches to research. Greenwood suggested that action research was a better alternative to the experimental method because it reflected the real constraints of nursing life (Greenwood 1984) and Melia felt that her qualitative study of student nurses enabled her subjects to 'tell it like it is' (Melia 1981). Goodman attempts to pour oil on these troubled waters by suggesting that it is a sign of nursing's increasing professional self-confidence that its researchers can adopt methods 'on the basis of their appropriateness for a given situation' and not on adherence to one approach. For her, qualitative and quantitative approaches 'lie along a continuum and do not occupy opposing camps' (Goodman 1989: 108). She ignores, however, the issue of academic and professional status and the political power that is associated with particular kinds of knowledge claim.

Leininger does not ignore such issues. Her strongly committed argument for nurses to embrace the previously considered 'second rate' qualitative research approaches is framed in terms of a political, professional and epistemological liberation. Her dedication to anthropologist Spradley in her *Qualitative Research Methods in Nursing* (Leininger 1985) emphasises the revolutionary claims of such an approach. Together with former colleague Spradley, she worked on 'fresh breakthroughs from traditional norms . . . spearheading new ways of generating knowledge . . . [with] pioneer zeal . . . [we] dared to be different . . . challenged dependency upon quantitative methodologies' (ibid.: v). If nursing is to become 'a fully recognised profession and discipline', she argues in the book's Preface, then there is a need for 'exploring and examining new and different types of research and theories to explicate the nature and essential features of nursing'. Qualitative methods reflect nursing's values. Leininger sets up a dualism between quantitative and qualitative approaches. The meanness of the characteristics credited to the former approach would find few champions. These attributes, drawn from her text, can be arranged as in Table 4.1.

If it might be expected, however, that Leininger turns away from the Enlightenment quest for the Truth of Nature; she goes on to privilege her approach with an ambitious metaphysical claim: 'Qualitative methodologies are, indeed the true and sound way to know the nature of human beings, their life-ways and health conditions' (Leininger 1985: xiii). Her justification for such methodologies is founded upon the same universal claims about the nature of human beings that she appears to reject in her summary of positivistic research. There are hints, indeed, that she wishes not to question but to intensify the

Table 4.1 Leininger's characteristics of quantitative and qualitative research

Quantitative approach	Qualitative approach
'people as reducible and measurable objects independent of historical cultural and social contexts'	'nursing's traditional values: personalised, intimate, holistic, human services'
'mainly statistical figures or data'	
'known in finite ways'	'elusive, vague unexplored nature of human care'
'reduced to parts or machine like operations'	
'sensual empirical data'	
'measurement, control and objectivity'	'knowing and understanding people'

Source: after Leininger 1985

Enlightenment's penetration into the human object of knowledge ever more deeply. This method, a convert is quoted as saying, 'has helped me to see the informant's world in ways I have never seen by quantitative methods' (ibid.). The anthropologist's term 'informant' is used but an informant reminds us of the underworld figure who is persuaded to betray their fellows to the authorities, revealing intimate and vital details. The language may be different, but the desire still appears to be for objectification and control. She urges nurses to move from 'scientific' legitimation to legitimation by association with the disciplines of anthropology and philosophy. Although presented in radical terms, authentification for her truth claims are still to be found within the Enlightenment science associated with the academic enterprise but with styles of inquiry found within different disciplines.

Others have echoed the same call, opposing on the one hand, a 'positivistic, natural science centred approach' to nursing knowledge and self-understanding which would keep nursing 'in the thrall of medicine' with, on the other, a 'genuinely holistic, person-centred approach' which is seen as the route to 'real professional autonomy' (Holmes 1990: 196). If science really is threatening nursing identity, it is attacking on two fronts; not just through doctors but, as Holmes, writing before the global introduction of 'market forces' into health care detects, from 'controlling authorities'. For him, the nursing profession has to decide whether

> the growing demand from controlling authorities for practice that is rational and scientifically defensible is reconcilable with the emergent belief that nursing is a human process in which the methods of measurement and quantification based on natural science epistemologies is inappropriate . . .
>
> (ibid.: 194)

Although Holmes' question is both appropriate and urgent, I would suggest that the science vs nursing knowledge dilemma is a false one for two reasons. First because of its totalising ambition, its assumption that one theoretical paradigm can be called upon to sufficiently explain human action and provide a knowledge base for the diverse range of activities undertaken by people accorded the title of 'nurse'. Second because of its striving for autonomy, a desire to act authoritatively, guided only by its own professional version of universal reason. This runs the danger of repeating the modern move attributed to medicine by seeking a theoretical and hence universalising (rather than an ethical or cultural) foundation for its actions and using this theoretical position to reduce and dominate the heterogeneity of practice.

Feminism, research and nursing

Some, from a feminist orientation, have grappled with the issues of power relationships within research or have looked at the construction of nursing knowledge and its relationship to 'scientific knowledge' from the point of view of such knowledge as women's knowledge. Hagell speaks of nurses as an 'epistemic community', a group with a particular frame of reference and a particular kind of knowledge that is 'based in part on their situation as women in a patriarchal society and in part as women involved in a specific gender-defined occupation – nursing, which is given little value in society' (Hagell 1989: 228).

She recounts the now familiar argument that nursing adopted the male-constructed values of (medico)scientific knowledge as its model for knowledge development in an attempt to gain autonomy and social status. In this way, in the area of knowledge, women have been colonised by men. She argues that caring is both the central activity and key value for nurses and she constitutes this caring orientation as diametrically opposed to scientific knowledge and values: 'science cannot conceptualise caring nor can caring be measured, only experienced' (ibid.: 231). Unfortunately, she argues, the adopting of such a scientific frame of knowledge has caused nursing's very essence to vanish. For her, if nurses (as women) can reclaim and revalue their experiential knowledge, and explore and define the 'nature of caring behaviours' then the profession's direction could be changed. The goal still seems to involve professional aggrandisement but its attainment is somehow made more likely by an exploration of caring knowledge.

The knowledge that is said to spring from experience, intimacy and caring appears idealised by Hagell and set in an untenable contrast to 'medicine and many other male dominated groups in the health field, which are based on the non-capacity to care' (Ashley 1980). Hagell erects a series of interlinked dualisms: 'caring/science, women/men and nursing/medicine'. At present, she argues, power belongs to the second category. Hagell privileges caring as an essence from which can flow both knowledge and power. If the nursing profession as a whole were to share her view, she suggests, knowledge and power would then fill the first category. However, the analysis repeats the structures it is analysing so that the preservation rather than the dissolving of these dualisms is vital for her critique and strategy. On closer inspection the borders between these dualisms dissolve; 'scientific' knowledge infects caring knowledge and vice versa, nursing and medicine become professional groupings with historically and culturally contingent borders rather than ontological givens, and gender in terms of values and behaviour, at least, becomes a continuum rather than an essentialised opposition. In other words, these are not fixed and mutually exclusive categories and to offer them as a philosophical foundation for a political strategy is to simplify and make static a shifting and contingent situation.

The claim that caring is nursing's unique essence is a source of vulnerability perhaps more than a strength (whether nurses have successfully defined this characteristic or not) if other groups effectively lay claim to it or if in society at large it remains an unvalued activity and orientation. A further problem seems to reside in a failure to see a tension between the desire, on the one hand, to improve the position of women as a whole, and on the other, to raise the occupational status of the nursing profession by claiming access to a particular kind of knowledge. Does this knowledge arise from the supposed biological given of gender, the social condition of women as unwaged or poorly paid carers, from systematically gained occupational and theoretical learning or from experience of the possible intimacy of caring? This desire to privilege one group of female carers is perhaps one of the most significant tensions beneath the whole issue of knowledge and nursing.

Others such as Salvage (1985) and Davies (1995) have attempted to recast the notion of professionalism to challenge its implicit gendered and elitist basis. Davies argues that traditional professional values are in some ways similar to those of bureaucracies in that they emphasise the adherence to generalisable principles of decision-making even though the encounter between the professional and his or her client appears to be highly individual. She also argues that it is precisely this kind of 'intellectual puzzle' approach to decision-making that it is suggested characterises the development of young boys while girls are said to draw upon more contextualised and personal awareness (Gilligan 1982). To the extent that these arguments are persuasive, they raise questions for a profession wishing to draw its authority from a theoretical knowledge base. Certain initiatives, such as the UK Royal College of Nursing's 'Value of Nursing' campaign attempted to reconstitute an alternative knowledge characterised by complexity, Benner's 'expert practice' (Benner 1984) and perhaps even intuition (Royal College of Nursing 1992).

Finally, Parker approaches the issue of nursing's role and identity in a way that possibly echoes environmental nursing models through the links that she forges between nursing and ecofeminism. For her, nurses have a unique access to the healing powers of nature that flow most readily through women (Parker 1993: 89). She evokes a picture of nursing as a humanising force in the dehumanising environment of technicist health care, a force that is fundamentally *embodied* in an increasingly theorised and abstract realm.

Knowledge, tradition, science and emancipation were powerful discourses drawn upon during the planning and introduction of the UK's reform of nurse education, Project 2000.

UK NURSING AND PROJECT 2000

In the mid-1980s, nursing's UKCC, itself only created in 1979, started work on devising a major reform of nursing education in the UK. That reform became known as Project 2000. It represented a significant, and almost successful, attempt to modernise nursing. The first key aim of the project was to change the nature of nurse education, from a system which was largely driven by the requirement to meet the workforce needs of the country's hospital and community-based health services to one that would expose its students (and educators) to the beneficial effects of mainstream education. In 1972 the Committee on Nursing chaired by Asa Briggs had criticised the neglected state of nursing in the NHS and strongly recommended a restructuring of the profession's regulatory bodies and a radical reform of nurse education (Committee on Nursing 1972). The former was achieved, although not without difficulty. Action on the latter was not taken until more than a decade later. 'Educational reform', wrote Celia Davies, 'was going to be the test-bed to establish whether the new grouping of the nursing professions could work together in a constructive fashion' (Davies 1995: 110). However, a number of contradictory forces added to the tension, the profession's own impatience for reform on the one side and the government's suspicion of the professions and intensified drives toward cost cutting in the public sector on the other.

The terms of reference of Project 2000 were

> to determine the education and training required in preparation for the professional practice of nursing, midwifery and health visiting in relation to the projected health care needs in the 1990s and beyond and to make recommendations.
>
> (UKCC 1986 cited by Davies 1995: 110)

The UKCC document argues the case for change, in part, by relying upon an assumption among its readers of a gloomy traditionalism within nursing. Change was relatively simply linked to progress. The characteristics of progress are signalled by more rational descriptions of nursing activity and increased talk of nursing in terms of the characteristics of professionals. The report noted that there had been

> wider developments, the use now of the nursing process and nursing models as analytical tools, the growing body of clinical research, and the development and consolidation of a model of primary nursing where an individual registered nurse is totally responsible and accountable for care.
>
> (UKCC 1986: 8)

The report also drew attention to a complex set of social changes that the period had witnessed together with their impact on health need and the pattern of health provision. A further factor marshalled to support the argument for change was the so-called demographic 'time bomb' ticking away in terms of a reducing pool of 18-year-olds, from which nursing traditionally recruited, against a background of an ageing general population.

Davies describes the context for the project; the series of amalgamations of over 600 schools of nursing in England in the early 1970s leaving less than 200 by the mid-1980s. Yet the period also witnessed the proliferation of educational courses for nurses, including degree courses, which were taught and awarded in association with a number of colleges and universities. Links into the higher education sector were clearly being forged in some areas well before Project 2000 recommended such action.

A consensus within the profession was said to be emerging. Educators felt the pressure of an ever growing curriculum while managers of the service were faced with the challenge of the increasing complexity of hospital work and a new emphasis on health care provided in the community. Wastage rates were also high; the service lost 30,000 nurses each year and a high proportion of student nurses left during training (Davies 1995). Only 65 per cent of those who started nurse training in England and Wales successfully reached the register (UKCC 1986). The Project committee held over 40 formal meetings with nurses and many more informal consultations. These meetings and other responses convinced the committee of a 'depth of frustration and dissatisfaction' within the profession at large.

In response, Project 2000 recommended an educational structure based on a year's training on a common foundation programme followed by training in a number of specialist branches. Enrolled nurse (EN) training, which was shorter than full registration, was to end but opportunities for retraining were to be provided. Students were to enjoy supernumerary status and to be funded by higher education grants rather than receive a wage from health authorities. The new system was expected to reduce wastage considerably and it was anticipated that 64–70 per cent of the nursing workforce would be trained.

The scheme, however, ran into serious problems. The government, while expressing commitment, declared the cost to be unacceptably high. It also disagreed about the cessation of EN training and argued that attention needed to be given to the recruitment of an untrained, support workforce. Funding was to allow only half the former students to be replaced with qualified nurses. Regional health authorities were asked to put forward submissions for schemes from institutions in a very short time-scale and, in the first year, only 13 of the 23 submissions were approved. By 1992, four years after the scheme's acceptance, four out of five nursing students were Project 2000 students while seventeen colleges were still running the old courses (Davies 1995).

A National Audit Office enquiry into the project's implementation identified the problems that the concurrent move to reduce public expenditure had caused it (National Audit Office 1992), while nurses themselves complained that the speed and confusion surrounding the implementation had affected recruitment into it.

However, a further, unanticipated and more far-reaching problem faced the scheme in the shape of the proposals to reform the NHS first announced in January 1989 (Department of Health 1989c). *Working for Patients: Working Paper 10* outlined the proposed arrangements for workforce training within the competitive NHS market. The amalgamated colleges and schools of nursing were to contract with local providers to meet the staffing and skill-mix needs that providers identified. In addition the National Vocational Qualifications scheme was to be extended. The opportunity for the educational aspirations of the nursing profession to escape its (100-year-old) thraldom to service needs and to a service faced with its own increasing financial constraints, became compromised in the very moment that it could have been realised. As Davies, one of the architects of Project 2000 concludes: 'The Project 2000 vision of a clearly demarcated and separate educational budget, managed by schools themselves, was being thoroughly overtaken by the new contract culture of the NHS' (Davies 1995: 123). It has indeed been overtaken. Today, in the late 1990s, education and training consortia translate the workforce requirements of local health care providers into contracts with local colleges of nursing and their purchasing power has recently been extended to include nursing courses at degree as well as diploma level.

THE NURSING PROFESSION AND THE NHS REFORMS

We can examine the formal response of the nursing profession to the rise of managerialism in two ways. First, we can look at its impact on nursing's place within the power structures of the NHS and second, we can consider how nursing leaders, including those in government posts, attempted to manage the interaction between the humanistic discourses associated with nursing and the more, perhaps, utilitarian discourses of managerialism.

The nursing 'voice' in health care

The NHS traditionally functioned with three separate management structures involving, respectively, administrators, doctors and nurses. Their contribution to consensus was, in theory, equal but in practice their power was asymmetrical. Successive waves of reforms shaped the management structures and influenced the level of opportunity for nurses to 'be heard in a way that doctors already were' (Owens and Glennerster 1990: 9). For example, the committee of inquiry that produced the Salmon Report (Ministry of Health 1966) recommended expanding the range of exclusively nursing management posts. A further reorganisation in 1974 extended this chain of command into newly formed layers of management at district, area and regional levels and marked the apotheosis of the model of separately managed professions. 'At long last' wrote two commentators, with possibly a touch of irony, 'nursing sat at the top table' (Strong and Robinson 1990: 19).

However, there were problems. The 'unwieldy conglomeration of diverse and, for the most part, relatively unskilled workers' (Strong and Robinson 1990: 19) that was the profession of nursing was challenged when it came to producing a significant body of credible managers. In addition, the new management structures did little to alter imbalances of power between the medical profession and administrators and nurses. This was an attempt to reshape an overall management structure on modern business lines while at the same time leaving unchallenged the structures of consensus. The evidence that this attempt was a failure lies in the enthusiasm with which, 10 years later, the Griffiths recommendations to end once and for all the rhetoric of consensus were greeted. However, they were not greeted eagerly by all. For Trevor Clay, then General Secretary of the Royal College of Nursing, general management 'undoubtedly wrecked the plans the profession had for changing its leadership profile' (Clay 1987: 57). Its ability to exercise control over its own destiny, at best tenuous, was severely curtailed. Clay caricatured the new general managers as wielding Filofaxes in which are inscribed a short list of priorities such as 'value for money' and others of an overwhelmingly financial nature. The advertising campaign mounted by the RCN in the national press also presented the public with simple, yet powerfully emotive, images; the male figure of the manager with pocket calculator set against various uniformed nurses including nurse archetype Florence Nightingale. The dualistic slogan 'a matter of life and death can become a matter of pounds and pence' indicating that the new managers were more interested in balancing books than caring for patients (Owens and Glennerster 1990), was paraphrased, nearly 12 years later, by a great many nurses in the present study.

Although the RCN stance may well have not encouraged nurses to apply for these posts, some nurses were appointed to general management positions. Many senior nurse managers, however, found themselves sidelined into 'advisory' posts or given undefined responsibility for 'quality' (Strong and Robinson 1990). As part of the 1991 NHS reforms, the government stipulated that Trust boards should include a director with a nursing background alongside medical and financial representation.

After initial opposition, the RCN attempted to influence the general management agenda rather than mount a frontal attack. In an attempt perhaps to woo this powerful group, an RCN 'Executive Trust Nurses Special Interest Group' was launched in January 1994 in the executive surroundings of London's Café Royale. A journal for nurses in management was launched in April 1994 by the RCN's publishing house. Presenting itself as a 'journal for nursing leaders', its first editorial described the nurse manager – and nursing's task – in the following way: 'It's about pragmatism. It's about helping the nursing profession to use its own massive resources to finally empower itself' (Naish 1994: 1).

Some nurses employed in the UK Department of Health promoted the idea that nurses could make good executives, arguing that they had the skills and brought nursing's characteristic human touch to the job. A study by the NHS Management Executive (NHSME 1992b) 18 months after the reforms, looked at the first year's experiences of 24 of the new nurse executive directors. The nurse executives felt that they had simultaneously established credibility for their role as manager and could act in a way that would promote the professional interests of nurses and advance something of that profession's value base. The report continually emphasised what appeared to be the considerable achievement of those with a nursing background being taken seriously outside the confines of the profession. The report's explicit purpose was to promote the role. A great many black-and-white photographs picture them in dynamic gestural poses, sometimes in the boardroom, or displaying apparently warm, human qualities in interactions with their staff or sitting beside patients in hospital beds. According to the report, the executives generally saw themselves as at the 'leading edge' of the profession's development.

A report by management consultants Newchurch (1995) gave the same message; that nurses could become involved, unproblematically, in senior management roles and that this represented a triumph for nursing rather than a source of confusion over its values.

Nursing and the Department of Health

During the period of the introduction of the NHS reforms a number of high-profile documents with relevance for nursing were released both by the Nursing Division of the Department of Health and the NHS Management Executive. Among these were *A Strategy for Nursing* (Department of Health 1989b), *A Vision for the Future* (Department of Health and National Health Service Management Executive 1993) and *New World, New Opportunities* (NHSME 1993). These documents represented a taking stock of the profession along with exhortations for its development. A particular approach to its development was apparent. The writers were keen to emphasise that the 'caring essence' of nursing should not be forgotten as the profession became increasingly sophisticated and modernised. In spite of this, nurses and their managers were urged to take on innovation and new language. Some innovations took the need for more careful resource use as their starting-point. Among these were the recommendation that value for money issues should be examined and attention given to eliminating waste of scarce resources. *A Vision for the Future*, in particular, adopted the phrase 'high-quality cost-effective' service with such ease and frequency that any suggestion that tension might exist between these two principles is effaced. (See the nurses' comments in Chapter 8 for their view of delivering 'quality' services in a situation of financial constraint.)

Other innovations related to this more indirectly. These included the development of outcome measures and a new emphasis on managerial and supervisory roles and aptitudes. The authors of *A Strategy for Nursing* saw the supervision of a range of less qualified or unqualified workers as an essential and increasing part of the nurse of the future's work. *New World, New Opportunities* emphasised the primary health care nurse's need to be skilled at 'self- and time management . . . patient care management . . . caseload management and team management' and its authors recommended that nurses should grasp opportunities for management roles and experience. In addition, a great deal of individual responsibility was expected of practitioners as they developed their own 'competence and confidence', supported generally not by line managers, but by more experienced colleagues acting in clinical supervision roles. Their accountability should be firmly goal-orientated. Alongside these visions were new attempts at 'partnership with users and their carers'. These took the form of the named nurse initiative, where each client or patient was told the name of one nurse who would assume responsibility for them throughout their period of care, and the stipulation that health care providers undertake satisfaction surveys among the users of their services.

'Nursing values' and the market

Early reflections from nurses less close to central government on the 1991 reforms were mixed. On the one hand, there was an apprehension. The RCN felt that the Department of Health's *Working for Patients: Working Paper 10* (1989c) 'undermined the principles and effectiveness of the NHS and placed at risk most of the progress that had been made since 1948' (Butler 1992: 60). Speaking at a management symposium in 1992, Trevor Clay commented that he found it hard to welcome a market structure 'which deliberately forces a competitive ethos on nurses'. He claimed that, by contrast, the values which underpin nursing are those of 'partnership, teamwork and collaboration' (*Nursing Standard News* 1992b). In the community health setting, where the field work of this study is located, virtually every aspect of the reforms was seen as a possible threat to nursing numbers or the status of nursing or both (Lowe 1990; North and Porter 1991; Prentice 1991; *Nursing Standard News* 1992a). For example, many community nurses, particularly health visitors, whose role is based upon preventive activities, expressed concerns not only about how to 'package their care attractively for GPs, self-governing Trusts, the NHS or even private organisations' but also how to quantify the 'unquantifiable' caring role of the nurse (Mason 1991). At other times, nurses were urged to be pragmatic in their approach to the reforms (*Nursing Times News* 1990) while others argued that central aspects of the reforms were entirely in line with community nurses' desire to provide high-quality, locally responsive services. For one writer in the popular nursing press, adopting a so-called 'marketing philosophy' (not quite a 'market philosophy') was a question not so much of survival but more of promoting some of nursing's client-centred values (Edwards 1994).

In addition, nursing discourse quite suddenly included the term 'productivity'. For example, Mary Daly, professional officer with the Health Visitors Association, the normally radical professional body representing health visitors, was quoted in that association's journal saying that 'official figures showed health visitor productivity has gone up' (*Health News* 1994). An RCN paper both highlighted apparently soaring nurse productivity, a measure derived from weighted hospital activity and cost data, while simultaneously questioning the discourse of productivity (Royal College of Nursing 1994). Drives for efficiency gave rise not just to a new discourse but to intensified scrutiny of the division of nursing labour. A number of often contradictory reports emerged from various sources making recommendations about methods for determining the most efficient (the cheapest feasible before particular measures of quality are affected) combination of levels of nursing skills (Buchan and Ball 1991; Audit Commission 1992; Car-Hill *et al.* 1992; Lightfoot *et al.* 1992; NHSME 1992a). The clinical grading exercise initiated in the 1980s is said to have facilitated this process by having 'produced a system which is essential to efficient management of nursing staff' (Holliday 1992: 19). In nursing research the current emphasis is on 'evidence based practice' (Ball 1991) and professional development emphasises the value of the nurse who can articulate and measure objectives and whose 'reflective practice' (Schön 1983), according to some managers interviewed in this research, includes reflections upon whether her activities could be carried out more efficiently by a lower grade of worker.

TODAY'S HEALTH SERVICE DISCOURSES

The 1970s 'oil crisis' coupled with 'world recession', the drastic reduction in power of the former Soviet Union along with the often televised 'fall' of communist regimes in many countries in Eastern Europe during the 1980s have led us to the political and cultural situation we find ourselves in today. The New Right's faith in economic rationalism and so-called market forces became coupled with 'consumerism' and a belief in managerialism. The scene has shifted decisively over the last 20 years. However, some have seen the recent health policy proposed by a Labour government in its 1997 White Paper (Department of Health 1997), for example, as an endorsement of their words of warning uttered in the early 1980s. Writing about the White Paper which proposed a model of clinical governance for the NHS, Christine Hancock, RCN General Secretary, referred to the 1984 'coccyx and humerus' campaign and commented:

> Ever since the [Griffiths] reforms, the NHS has been dogged by a culture of general management. It's a culture that says if you can manage an engineering factory, then you can also manage a hospital or a community health service. Undoubtedly there are some transferable skills but, ultimately, health care doesn't work like an engineering firm. People aren't machines. Even general managers now realise that you need people in charge who understand the process of health care. People like nurses.
>
> (Hancock 1998: 20)

It is hard to say how far the change of government in the UK in 1997 has brought in a significant change of ethos. So far, the promise of the new primary care groups, which are to be given responsibility for commissioning local primary care services, has not effected a shift in the established power balance between doctors and nurses. It is unclear how far the proposed clinical governance will restore to the clinical professions the influence that they may have had before the introduction of general management.

Nevertheless, today's health care discourses emphasise, in one way or another, the more efficient use of limited resources. This is its legitimised language which those seeking influence in health care ignore at their peril. It is then little surprise to find nursing discourse speaking, for example, of the need for the development of 'outcome measures' (Alexander *et al.* 1993; Zlotnick and Gould 1993) and 'evidence-based practice' (Ball 1991).

Nursing and evidence-based practice

As part of its identity and power structure, any professional group seeks to establish a unique body of knowledge. This involves first, either implicitly or explicitly identifying what counts as a valid knowledge claim, and second, placing the activity of its members into a particular context, be it moral or scientific. The rise of the 'evidence-based' movements in the 1990s has provided the clinical professions with opportunities for intensified identity and for re-establishing power in the face of increases in lay knowledge and threats from managerial control. Nursing's established clinical effectiveness programmes meant that many nurses were well prepared for this new movement. However, clinical effectiveness/EBM creates a mainstream of credible health care from which no practitioner or professional group dare be excluded. To not fit in is to risk being consigned to a denigrated position without seriousness, credibility, morality, future or funding. Alongside a confidence its rise stirred nursing's fears of marginalisation: 'In support of nurses' involvement in clinical effectiveness, Kitson (1997) urged nurses to identify evidence to justify their practice and suggested that this is how they will be accepted as 'players' within the 'evidence-based medicine/clinical effectiveness movement' (McClarey and Duff 1997: 33).

Of course, in one sense, effectiveness and outcomes are appropriate things to be talking about. What is of interest is the way that this talk has become incorporated within, or one might say has colonised, the construction of 'professional development'. One aim, at least, of professional development is the nurse who can articulate her objectives, demonstrate and measure her impact using particular criteria, possibly legitimised by managers (Bloomfield *et al.* 1992), can manage a team of lesser skilled workers, and who is constantly questioning whether the same effect can be achieved more efficiently (Johns 1995). This discourse may take on the language of professional development but this tends to mask its contingent nature as a response to particular economic circumstances, suggesting that such an approach is desirable in an acontextual way.

To summarise, I would suggest that nursing leaders have continually reshaped discourse about the profession – the way it is talked about and how it is valued

– in response to changing discourses in society at large, for example discourses of morality, science, feminism, consumerism and most recently economic rationalism. These discourses have also influenced nursing education and research issues. Such discourses often have functioned in a way that has marginalised particular values or groups within nursing. Chapter 8, which presents the comments of the nurses involved in this research, gives voice to some of those 'disqualified knowledges'.

But even apart from the perhaps relatively lonely voices of nurses involved in this research, it would be a mistake, as I mentioned at the outset, to understand nursing as having one voice and being engaged in one project. However, some discursive projects can be seen as achieving ascendance at particular moments in history.

The next chapters will go on to explore the words of managers and nurses in the light of issues of claims to knowledge, the basis of legitimacy and power.

5 The origins of the texts: management interviews and nursing questionnaires

It's just before 9 on a Monday morning and the atmosphere is rather edgy, the start of another week. PA to the Chief Exec comes in. 'I think the whole issue has been misunderstood – he wanted to make it easy not difficult . . . ' she is saying to the Finance Director. For some reason the FD goes off to see the Director of Nursing Practice. From the room where I am waiting I hear (but don't see) the Chief Exec arrive. I hear him say to his secretary as he is walking into his office, 'Had a good weekend?' then disappears. His staff ring through to him to tell him I am here. His PA refers to him by his first name. Before me, the Finance Director (who has managed to squeeze in to see him) comes out of his office still looking rather grim. I am waiting in the Chairman's simple but neat office, too neat to be true. On the wall are three graphs, one displaying a falling line entitled 'Waiting Lists' and another with a steadily rising line called '[Trust name] Contracts' and another showing similarly rising 'Hospital Separations'.

(Author's field notes)

The initial aims of the fifty interviews that I carried out with the new Trust managers were to learn about their strategies, employment practices and views about the recent NHS legislation. After a while I began to wonder whether thinking of these managers as creators of strategies was the best way of thinking about their part in these brave new reforms. Perhaps this was to take these notions of potency or agency, the reforms' rhetoric of freedom and independence too seriously, too much at face value. I began to wonder whether these managers, like the nurses they managed, the patients that were treated and the many researchers, like me, who researched them, were caught up in a drama that was an outworking of an ideology or a 'mood'. Some of its inspiration lay in the 'freedom to be entrepreneurial' celebrated by the Thatcher Conservative government. Other ancestors were the more distant philosophical moments in Europe's history that emphasised the power of human reason to grant a limitless autonomy to human thought and action. Some managers rose to the challenge with more accomplishment than others.

As I outlined in Chapter 1, a longitudinal research study was undertaken to examine the impact of the NHS 1991 reforms upon community health services. A sample of four first wave NHS Trusts which had responsibility for community nursing services were recruited to the research. In one of the areas served by the

Trust which I have called Optimist Community Health Trust, health visitors, who play, or potentially play, an important preventative community nursing role, were employed by an acute hospital Trust within a child health directorate. They were included in the study along with their own small team of managers and I have designated their organisation as Brick-built Hospital Trust. The study initially, therefore, went into five separate organisations.

Along with these interviews, the study comprised three rounds of questionnaires to the nursing workforce assessing their job satisfaction. I give more details of this in Chapter 8. This questionnaire component of the study started in April 1991 and was repeated once in each of the two subsequent years. In order to elicit management views and responses to the reforms, it was decided to interview a range of managers, taken from different levels within each of the organisations under study, at similar yearly intervals. However, these interviews started some months after the questionnaire surveys, in 1992, and the last round was completed in 1994. This delay was due to the constraints of the size of the research team with one person carrying out the field work, data entry, report writing and most of the clerical duties. A serendipitous outcome was that it was possible to ask managers to respond to some of the results of the satisfaction survey of their staff. The research was designed for it to be possible to compare the views of managers in the different organisations, managers with different backgrounds, for example, administrative, medical or nursing, managers at different levels in the same organisation as well as their views over time. The management structure and size of the Trusts varied. Of the 29 managers involved five were men.

Initially a perhaps naive assumption was made in the research unit that various 'management styles' could be identified within the study and linked to differing levels of workforce job satisfaction that might emerge. In practice, the situation quickly proved far too complex for such lines of cause and effect to be drawn.

The study gave rise to different types of 'data', the short and often passionate comments written by nurses on the questionnaires, their other utterances noted during Trust meetings that I attended, field notes and impressions and the longer transcripts of the interviews. Certain types of comparison between them would clearly be inappropriate. However, for my purposes, a distinction between the rhetoric of foundational values to which each group made appeal in the achievement of its subjectivity could be made, in spite of the fact that the nurses' texts were short written comments and the managers' were the product of more expansive interviews.

At the time scheduled for the interviews in one of the Trusts, which I designate Absolute Trust, its management team was considering withdrawing from the study after senior managers had received the research unit's confidential report of its workforce's job satisfaction during the study's first year. Nurses' satisfaction was low and later turned out to be by far the lowest in the study. Absolute Trust managers suggested that the research had a 'hidden agenda' to present NHS Trusts in a poor light and the location of the research unit within a nursing trade union contributed to this suspicion. Interviews that I had arranged with its ten locality managers were cancelled by the Trust's senior management, who offered instead one group interview with all of these locality managers together with the nurse executive and in the presence of a manager from their personnel department. This interview was carried out, although the group declined my request to tape record the meeting. I have not included an analysis of this session here, although it might have made an interesting study of the managed encounter. In the event, and after four months of non-response to our correspondence, the Trust's management informed us that it was withdrawing from the study because it was undertaking its own internal communication study and therefore did not need to participate further. Perhaps job satisfaction and this arguably insecure, closed management style might, after all, be linked. In the first year, I carried out 23 interviews with managers from across the three remaining Trusts.

For the second year of interviews, undertaken during the summer of 1993, I selected a sub-sample of two managers from each Trust from an analysis of the first-year transcripts. One manager was chosen from each Trust as appearing to adopt a style of talk generally representative of a 'mainstream' view in that Trust while another was chosen who, in some way, used atypical language to express atypical views for the Trust, or to put it another way, who appeared troubled about the 'mainstream' identity worked at by the majority of the organisation's managers. For example, in a Trust where there was much emphasis on explicit definitions and quantification of the effect of nursing work, one manager went to great pains to express concern that the less tangible aspects of nursing may be forgotten. Sampling in this fashion, it was possible to gain access to a wide range of views in the most economical way.

The third-year interviews were carried out between March and October 1994, using the same sampling approach as the first year. Because of restructuring within the Trusts, 21 instead of 23 interviews were carried out. A summary of the interviews carried out is given in Table 5.1. The job titles of the managers reflect different organisational structures.

Table 5.1 Interview timetable: all years

Optimist Community Health Trust	Brick-built Hospital Trust	Sceptical Health Services Trust	Pragmatic Community Health Services
Year 1: April – September 1992			
Chief executive	Senior manager – health visiting 1	**Chief executive**	**Chief executive**
Nurse executive	and senior manager – health visiting	**Nurse executive**	**Nurse executive**
Nurse advisor	2 together	Director of Primary Care Directorate	Director of local services

continued

Table 5.1 continued

Locality manager 1 Locality manager 2 Locality manager 3 Locality manager 4	**Assistant director of Primary Care Directorate**		Nurse advisor Locality manager
		Locality manager 1 Locality manager 2 Locality manager 3 Locality manager 4	Neighbourhood manager 1 Neighbourhood manager 2 (chosen at random from 11 neighbourhood managers)

Year 2: May – September 1993

Nurse executive	Senior manager – health visiting 1	Locality manager 1 Locality manager 3	**Nurse executive** Nurse advisor

Year 3: March – October 1994

Chief executive **Nurse executive** Locality manager 1 Locality manager 2 Locality manager 4	Senior manager – health visiting together with 3 locality managers – health visiting*	**Chief executive** **Nurse executive** Director of clinical services (was previously director of Primary Care Directorate) **Director of Primary Care Directorate** (was previously Assistant director of Primary Care Directorate) Locality manager 1 Locality manager 2 Locality manager 3 Locality manager 4 (new in post)	**Chief executive** **Nurse executive** Director of local services **Nurse advisor*** (retiring) Neighbourhood manager 1 **Neighbourhood manager 7*** (not previously interviewed) Neighbourhood manager 8 (last two purposively sampled and not previously interviewed)

* 'Unconverted' managers

Note: Absolute Trust withdrew after the first year of the study. The one group interview undertaken in this organisation is not included in the analysis

The interviews

These semi-structured interviews lasted approximately 50 minutes each and were tape recorded and transcribed in full either by myself or by an audiotypist contracted to the research unit. The questions addressed were extremely wide-ranging and involved personal background and employment issues which might reveal differences over time and between Trusts such as numbers employed, nursing skill-mix, conditions of employment and in-service training. There were also questions concerning information systems, management structure, policies and practices for communication within the organisation, relationships with other organisations such as the major purchaser of its services (the Health Authority or Commission), social service departments and general practitioners, and questions about contracting, the difference Trust status had made to individual managers, management qualifications and views about the nursing profession and its future. Interview transcripts were initially coded with the aid of The Ethnograph V. 3.0 (Seidel 1988) computer software.

For the purposes of this study which is concerned with close textual analysis rather than a summary of content, I decided to concentrate attention upon nineteen interviews. These interviews are indicated in bold type in Table 5.1. They comprise interviews carried out with nine individuals and one small group interview with a team of three managers of health visitors. Of this sample two of the twelve managers were men. The individuals include all three nurse executives, all three chief executives and one senior community manager from the Trust where community nurses were managed in a separate directorate. These people were chosen because of their leading positions in their organisations. Although it is possible to argue for a reading of the texts of even the highly committed that includes some ambivalence regarding the political origins and implementation of the reforms, these individuals were likely to present the 'official' views of the organisation. In a similar fashion to the selection of a small sub-sample of managers that I described above, certain interviews with managers who expressed clearly hesitant views about the reforms and certain aspects of their organisations, or who were groping for another language, or caught uneasily between two (or more) discourses, were also selected for close analysis. These were a nurse adviser and a locality manager from one of the Trusts and the small management team of three health visitors from another Trust. Interviews with 'unconverted' managers are indicated by asterisks in Table 5.1.

Analysis of this smaller sample of nineteen interviews was greatly helped by the use of another, more flexible, computer program, NUD•IST (Richards and Richards 1994). A range of differences that were expected at the outset of the research between the discourse of, for example, executives with nursing and those with administrative backgrounds, between the male and female managers and between the three years of the study were, in practice, hard to detect with any confidence. Differences between the organisations were more obvious, though rarely startling. The managers of Optimist Community Health Trust and Pragmatic Health Services appeared to adopt a more charismatic style of managerial discourse (Rafferty 1993b) and spoke of a more innovative approach to the organisation of care delivery while management talk in Sceptical Health Services Trust tended to feature disappointment that the reforms had failed to deliver an expected range of freedoms and attention to remedial organisational action. Quotations presented in the following chapters identify the Trust and the job title of the speaker. They do not identify the year of the comment unless it is important for a specific point of argument. Although the content of managers' arguments changed during the course of the study, the structures and strategies of their argumentation did not appear to.

An approach to the texts

As explorations of the literature that I introduced in Chapters 2 and 3 progressed, it became clear that the analysis of the interviews and questionnaire comments could be taken in an entirely different direction to that of the original purposes of the RCN research. Rather than concentrate on the information contained in the answers to the questions, on the intentional 'meaning' of those interviewed, I sensed that an analysis of the language that flowed through their arguments almost as if it had independent existence of its own, might provide some knowledge of the discourses at work in contemporary UK health care, and of the identities made available to contemporary health care managers. Using the social medium of language, social actors participate in the meanings supplied by language so that it is not precise to say that an 'I' speaks (Heckman 1986).

Analysis was facilitated by becoming familiar with the content of the texts over the period of producing RCN reports. In the case of the first-year management interviews this involved returning to the texts for up to three years. I discarded an initial coding frame based upon the topics discussed by the speaker used in the RCN study for the purposes of this analysis.

Examples of the possibilities of this approach to analysis have been given in Chapter 3. Overall this analysis concentrates on the *textuality* of the data by adopting some of the practices of discourse analysis alongside the more literary and philosophical approach associated with deconstruction. It examines the way discursive effects are achieved by looking at the strategies and structures of discourse. Analysis includes an alertness to the following:

* descriptions and examples of the achievement of various kinds of rationality at work such as financial rationality;
* the creation of the 'objects' of discourse such as a 'new technocratic nurse';
* the adopting of various subject positions;
* the work of metaphor and the part it plays in the construction of argument;
* dualism in argument;
* the reifying of autonomy.

These areas, particularly those relating to types of rationality, knowledge and autonomy, were chosen for investigation because they appeared to have a place within the notion of modernity critiqued by the writers reviewed in Chapter 2.

Table 5.2 represents the final state of the coding categories devised during the use of the NUD•IST program in the textual analysis for this study. NUD•IST allows the creation of a taxonomy of categories, which it refers to as indexing *categories*, that can be linked to certain passages in the texts, and presents them graphically as an inverted tree-like diagram. While envisaging indexing categories in hierarchical relationships is potentially limiting because it may shape (possibly unconsciously) the process of thinking about the texts, it proved to be a good enough, pragmatic framework within which to organise the beginning of analysis. Indeed, the imposition of categories *at all* upon these texts, as upon any other object of inquiry, reduces their heterogeneity as the inquirer asks, in this case, whether any given passage falls either inside or outside the criteria of any particular category. Table 5.2 includes a brief definition of each category. The principal categories are shown in bold type; subcategories in plain type, an oblique stroke representing a subcategory.

Table 5.2 Indexing categories used in the analysis of texts

Rhetoric
Definition: rhetorical effects; alliteration, repetition, irony, 'high rhetoric', punning, dialogue

Subject position
Definition: the speaker strikes a subject position

Subject position/public interest
Definition: subject position adopted 'responsiveness to the public'

Subject position/visionary
Definition: subject position adopted of visionary

Subject position/therapist
Definition: acting in the best interest of staff's desires and welfare

Subject position/democrat
Definition: subject position as open, devolving, democratic leader

Subject position/revolutionary
Definition: working against traditions and traditionalists

Subject position/risk-taker
Definition: the speaker describes themselves or their actions as risk-taking

Subject position/balancer
Definition: 1. finds from text search for 'balance'; 2. other references to this idea

Subject position/professional
Definition: a professional discourse, perhaps set against something else

Parasite
Definition: the exclusion of a 'special case' as parasitic upon a mainstream case

Dualism
Definition: contains a whole or part dualism, either part of a whole system or a single occurrence

Rational
Definition: the parent of all types of rationality in the study

Table 5.2 continued

Rational/measurement
Definition: a type of rationality that is to do with measurement sometimes as opposed to 'subjective' impressions

Rational/financial
Definition: financial rationality as an ontological given

Rational/surveillance
Definition: watching/measuring/shaping by holding accountable what staff are doing

Rational/thinking
Definition: rational thinking as opposed to irrationality, e.g. fear, tradition

Rational/'computer'
Definition: search for 'computer', how people talked about this

Object
Definition: an instance of an 'object' created by a discourse

Object/stress
Definition: stress among staff or managers

Object/modern world
Definition: an appeal to modernity, the new or to today's world, triumphalism, technology

Object/dead wood
Definition: the people in an organisation who are not seen to be performing adequately

Object/good worker
Definition: talk of the group or individual worker who is progressive/ shares the management ethos

Object/traditional nurse
Definition: the nurse who is not corporate, rational, but who is individualistic, unquestioning, etc.

Metaphor
Definition: a piece of text that uses metaphor: the following categories

Metaphor/visual 1
Definition: visual metaphors part 1 looking (at), perspective, overview

Metaphor/visual 1/looking
Definition: text searches from, look(ing) overview and perspective

Metaphor/not visual
Definition: a huge range of metaphors that are not visual metaphors

Metaphor/boardroom
Definition: business/managerial world metaphors

Metaphor/boardroom/'agenda'
Definition: 'agenda' used metaphorically

Metaphor/boardroom/'business'
Definition: search for 'business'

Autonomy
Definition: where autonomous action is desired, claimed for the organisation or individuals

'Tradition'
Definition: results of a text search for 'tradition' plus talk of traditionalism

Transcript or speech . . . or text?

The subject of analysis and what the reader now approaches is not 'the speech itself' but the written word now presented out of the context of the interviews. Derrida's challenge to the view that writing is unoriginal, unreliable, open to misinterpretation and 'parasitic' on the original utterance has already been summarised (see Chapter 2, pp. 39–44). The very iterability that is at the heart of language means that, in a sense, the interviews do not provide the original context for the utterances that appear there. The words of the managers and the written words of the nurses can be understood as a continuous stream of quotations, each placed in a different context to its previous appearance. (What is striking about their words, as will be seen, is their *un*originality.) Nevertheless, the characteristics of spoken language have a certain charm, the appearance of which poets and playwrights have been at pains to contrive since the beginning of literary recording. It is therefore for this sentimental reason, rather than through any desire for naturalism that I have resisted the temptation to improve the grammar of the spoken language, to cut redundant phrases, hesitations, false starts or in other ways sanitise the texts for their presentation here. This has not been without its problems. Part of the RCN research involved presenting participants with intended quotations before their inclusion in reports. This was done so that unnoticed identifying information might be removed. Some managers, clearly sensitive to issues of representation, at that stage insisted that repetitious or otherwise unattractive sections be altered. 'It makes me sound silly. . . . I say "actually" 100 times. . . . I must have had a word of the week and that week it was "actually"' (from telephone conversation with a chief executive). Partly to maintain the goodwill of participants and partly because of the broader aims of the RCN project, these wishes were usually acceded to. However, here the texts are presented in unexpurgated form. The one convention followed has been the introduction of sentence-like structures, i.e. the insertion of punctuation and sometimes this has involved difficult judgements at the transcribing stage. Even this has necessarily imposed a structure on the texts.

IMPRESSIONS OF THE MANAGERS AND THEIR ORGANISATIONS

Before the main part of the analysis, I include two vignettes taken from field notes made during the research. They evoke something of the atmosphere within the organisations under study, with their mixture of activity, conscious self-presentation, excitement and suspicion. These characteristics reflect not only the ambience of these three organisations but, perhaps the whole atmosphere within the UK health service in the immediate wake of the reforms.

6th August 1992 At Pragmatic Community Health Services – asked to wait in the chairman's office by bright PA to the chief exec [CEO]. It occurs to me that the chairman's role is to provide a waiting room facility for the CEO. Like in Sceptical Health Services Trust, this office is like a theatre set – VERY neat, an 'Our Corporate Contract' chart from the Regional Health Authority pinned on the notice board, a small table with neatly fanned back numbers of *Health Service Journal* and back copies of the local trust publicity also 1 copy (only) of the yearly report which PA suggested 'I might like to read' while I was waiting. Up above, half of a bookshelf of management books:

In Search of Excellence
Personnel Management
Daring to Connect
When Giants Learn To Dance
Statistics for Business
A Woman in Your Own Right (strange as the chair is a man)

. . . and some others.

Afterwards: The interview was disappointing. The CEO kept me waiting so that we had little time to develop a conversation. She said there had been 'a crisis' (there is always a crisis) and as I was leaving she was already onto a different planet, dealing with her PA and secretary. I had the feeling she wasn't terribly into this. Before she agreed to be taped, she asked whether she could see the interview schedule and looked it through briefly. I had the feeling she was looking for a particular, probably controversial topic which clearly she didn't find. What ever it was, I should have been asking it.

February 1993 I am sitting outside the office where they [Director of Nursing and locality managers] are meeting, waiting to be asked in. Mostly it's quiet but there are occasional bursts of laughter. Eventually the Director of Nursing [DO] comes out. We shake hands and he asks me in. Three of the four locality managers are sitting round a small table; the fourth locality manager, the only man, has sent his female assistant so the DO is the only man. He is chairing this meeting. I have met three of the locality managers before and am surprised that these normally vocal people are so quiet here. It's a planning meeting and the DO comes up with plans that are breathtaking with their simple rationality: 'With our planned admission programme we can actually match our skill-mix on duty at any time to the expected workload.' They are all into it, but he is clearly best at it or at least the most articulate. The others are like a chorus, uttering supporting exclamations or observations of how irrational nurses are: 'Just because Florence Nightingale made beds in the morning means we've got to do it like that' (irony) or 'Nurses are terrible at time-management.' One locality manager who was assistant when I last met her is in her late fifties. (Later, reading between the lines of her secretary's careful comment to me, I learnt that she became seriously ill.) I feel she is a late convert to all this and, like religious converts, seems to continually celebrate her conversion with testimonies of her former life: 'We used to be saying that we were overworked forty years ago and they're still complaining about it now!' The DO comes in with 'What we ought to do is, if they *don't* complain, take staff away because they must have too many'. I thought he was making a joke, but nobody is laughing.

The next chapter offers an analysis of various forms of rationality in the texts. Chapter 7 concentrates upon accounts of subject positions adopted within the texts, the objects of discourse and constructions of autonomy and tradition. As an exploratory tool, the discourse of those managers unconvinced about the reforms has generally been compared to that of the managers who were committed to using them. Chapter 8 considers the texts of nurses' comments.

6 The interviews part I: discourses of rationality

RGM: I went to see Roy Griffiths in his office at Sainsbury's and while I was talking to him, his secretary handed him a piece of paper. He looked at it and said 'OK'. I asked him, 'What do you mean, "OK"?' and he said, 'My organisation is OK today'. It turned out he had just six measures on that piece of paper and from those he could tell what the state of Sainsbury's health had been the day before; things like the amount of money taken yesterday, the freshness quotient – the amount of stuff still on the shelves – the proportion of staff on duty, and so on.

(Strong and Robinson 1990: 81)

An inspector arriving unexpectedly at the centre of the Panopticon will be able to judge at a glance, without anything being concealed from him, how the entire establishment is functioning.

(Foucault 1977: 204)

TYPES OF RATIONALITY

A characteristic of modernity is that it describes itself as replacing tradition with rational thinking and activity, subduing 'nature and myth' so that nothing remains outside, 'because the mere idea of outsidedness is the very source of fear' (Adorno and Horkheimer 1996: 201). For example, Weber saw bureaucracies as mechanisms and embodiments of impersonality, impartiality and functionality in contrast – and such definitions are always dependent upon some act of exclusion – to relationships based on individual privileges and bestowal of favour which were said to characterise traditional structures. 'Above all there is a separation of the public world of rationality and efficiency from the private sphere of emotional and personal life' (Pringle 1988: 86). The managers in this study spoke about their approach in a way that often contrasted aspects of rationality with a previous or more primitive state that they encountered within their organisations. Indeed, it might be ventured that the two gifts they came bearing were culture and rationality; culture whether of 'risk-taking' or of 'valuing one's workers', serving the ends of rationality. However, a discussion of ultimate purposes is premature. The traditional society that the managers came to reform was manifest in the ancient and arcane secrets at the heart of the professions, knowledge that afforded them a privilege almost anachronistic in an age of reason. Paradoxically, medicine and, during particular stages in its history, nursing, have presented themselves in the same light, as bearers of the rationality of science. Yet a subsequent wave of rationality, taking as its point of reference financial control, has overtaken them and made them seem almost superstitious by contrast. The second tradition was of fear, ignorance and superstition embodied and traditionally associated with the womanly arts (Jordanova 1989), one of whose descendants in the modern world is the occupation of nursing. The third tradition is also associated with women; that of the realm of emotions and of the home, the site and crucible of so much emotional work. All these traditions are pushed to the margins and excluded by managerial discourse.

It can be useful to talk about four aspects of such rationality: the rationality of measurement, the rationality of finance as an ontological given, the rationality of surveillance and control, and a more overarching rationality that perhaps can only exist, be discussed and made visible when contrasted, as the managers did, with another mode of being such as fear, a partial picture, lack of objectivity, emotion, partiality. These are the modes of rationality referred to in the interviews.

MEASURING THE MARIGOLD

Managerialism seems to have rediscovered Newton's practice of repeated observation and the keeping of meticulous records. During the interviews it emerged that a major project in each Trust was the establishment of systems of scrutiny of activity and the chronicling of the results. This was presented as a new dawn for the NHS. To know what doctors and nurses were doing, to truly discern the nature and health of the organisation, required measurement of increasing sophistication. The metaphors associated with this discernment, this deep investigation were overwhelmingly visual: 'we are looking at . . . '. As knowledge became increasingly synonymous with information which was stored electronically in endless and indifferent successions of zeros and ones, measurement became a symbol of objectivity, of a metaphysical pursuit of the trustworthy and the real. Numerical information represented a repositioning of language-dependent knowledge, number being the 'canon of the Enlightenment' as Adorno and Horkheimer argued. Numbers can make 'the dissimilar comparable by reducing it to abstract quantities' (Adorno and Horkheimer 1979). Yet however strenuously this abstraction was aimed at and asserted, at the heart of such practices inevitably lay ultimately subjective and interested decisions. Whose and which activities should be recorded? How should they be represented and how can they be translated into performance, reward and discipline? What forces shall be allowed to remain invisible? What financial fears and incentives, aspirations, scores to settle and power to assert lurked at the borders of such an apparently lucid project? The almost Socratic dialectical encounter between clear reason and artful sophistry staged at moments by the managers can be dissolved into a much more evenly matched quest for persuasion. The interviews demonstrated not so much the manager's command of verifiable information as their skill at the art of persuasion.

The reforms, particularly in their early months, were highly politically contentious and a subject for constant media scrutiny. Within the Trusts being studied many workers were suspicious of their management's intentions and deeply opposed to the notion of an internal market. For some, memories of the introduction of general management were still bitter and the latest reforms represented a deepening of an unacceptable ethos of commercialism. Managers told how their staff were being unnecessarily disturbed by unfounded media stories which they saw as sometimes blatantly political in intent. This was one reason that they gave for placing a great deal of emphasis on 'openness of communication' within their organisations. Openness included promulgating 'information' about the Trust's activities. Senior managers would regularly carry out 'lecture tours' of staff bases, or 'road shows' partly to counteract politically motivated misinformation with hard data.

> 'The chief exec. goes on almost a lecture tour, starting early April to actually go out and tell people [staff] how we are doing, how we did last year, how many patients we saw, how that was better than the year before, what our financial position was at the end of the year, so that people actually know how the Trust did, so it's first hand, rather than sort of a jaded documentary on Channel Four.'
>
> (nurse executive, Optimist Community Health Trust)

Here the numerical and financial are set against the 'jaded' documentary, providing 'first-hand', verifiable knowledge. Patient throughput and financial information, interesting and important as they are, are partial yet are equated with the whole health of the Trust, 'how we are doing . . . actually know how the Trust did'. Evidence of increasing throughput was often on display during the research as ascending lines on graphs on the walls of the Trust chair's offices that I waited in.

Measurement and the numerical appeared to offer a new breakthrough or a rediscovery, a new language that all needed to learn in order to be taken seriously. The personal claim, unsupported by even rudimentary counting could be discounted as suspect, little short of nagging, ludicrous:

> 'I met the Day Ward Sister on my rounds and she was on about staffing and I said "you have evidence here of that[?]" and she'd done no record of patient dependency.'
>
> (nurse executive, Sceptical Health Services Trust)

Valid knowledge therefore contains an assurance of the impartial, a reference to some disembodied procedure or criteria.

As in Weber's bureaucracies, privilege is bestowed through the impartial application of rules. Rational measurement was described as providing the just and appropriate means of achieving this. For a manager committed to performance-related rewards as a motivator for the workforce, this meant turning to a range of 'indicators', which could be combined and used as the basis for bonuses.

> 'But of course I also think we are looking at team reward as well rather than individual reward, for if the team consistently achieve a high quality of patient satisfaction and whatever, you know there's lots of indications you could use, maybe I could give bonuses for that and again, that might not be cash, it might be something else. It might be a dinner, I don't know . . . '
>
> (nurse executive, Optimist Community Health Trust)

The interpretation of 'indicators' is wide.

> 'I mean, we have a low turnover rate and I think that's a good indicator when people are fairly, one of the indicators, of people being satisfied.'
>
> (nurse executive, Optimist Community Health Trust)

It is possible to ask whether turnover is more indicative of satisfaction, or high unemployment and lack of alternative nursing employment in a rural area.

Measurement could also be focused, and in apparently and authoritatively minute detail, upon the patient and his or her 'need' for care by a nurse with a particular level of qualification. The dependency of the patient is, in a sense, separated from the patient him or herself so that it can be visually examined, set alongside and compared with the dependency of a range of others. This is Foucault's normalising practice at work (Foucault 1977). The process of fitting expenditure to dependency is described in the following passage as so supremely rational that the nurses involved are drawn into the process and appear *themselves* to make these decisions. The context of the operation is set by the scientific 'analysis' and the use of the computer to reveal knowledge previously hidden. They have 'actually looked' for the first time. This context allows the speaker to describe the cheaper and less qualified worker subsequently employed as 'a good nurse to undertake the work':

> 'Now when we've analysed the work that was being done, we've actually looked at what needed to be done by trained nurses and not by the nurse . . . by actually printing out the caseload, looking at the work with the nurses and when we've needed to replace a member of staff we've actually realised that a staff nurse, or an enrolled nurse, would actually provide a good nurse to undertake the work that could be done.'
>
> (community manager, Sceptical Health Services Trust)

Having established aggregated dependency, the computer, after appropriate expenditure can go on to make visible the actual 'quality' of the resulting care delivered:

> 'We've spent a lot of money on the community, physical side of the business, developing an information system that will collect information and we're really still at the stage of trying to implement that community system, which is the foundation to actually being able to report on quality outcomes and until that's in place it's going to be quite difficult to get any meaningful information.'
>
> (chief executive, Optimist Community Health Trust)

As mentioned earlier, senior managers often presented their organisations to various groups (see p. 97). The detail with which the chief executive quoted below was able to speak would give a strong impression of intimate knowledge as well as finely tuned control, yet again this impression of being able to encapsulate the well-being of the organisation is achieved through numerical, and in this case, financially detailed calculation. It is here, towards these financial accounts that all these measurements point and have their meaning:

> 'We had our AGM on Tuesday this week and the slides I showed, showed that we had brought our unit cost down each year by about 50 pence per case so it's gone down to an average of about £18.50, £18.52 to be precise, I remember it, to £17.40 or £17.50, so it's gone £18.50, £18.00, £17.50 and that's a lot of money across thirty odd thousand cases.'
>
> (chief executive, Sceptical Health Services Trust)

Having convinced an audience of the accuracy of his ability to measure, by being 'precise' down to the nearest two pence, this manager can emphasise his point by switching to the rhetoric of grand imprecision by ending with 'that's a lot of money across thirty odd thousand cases.'

In a sense the contracting between purchaser and provider which was at the heart of the reforms provided a rationale for this new emphasis on measurement and measurability but contractual agreements did not always appear to be entirely numerically based. The repeated 'evidence' in the reading by a community manager from a 'quality' document below and the recital of the 'monitoring' and 'reports that . . . demonstrate' lead inevitably to numerically presented 'evidence'. The intention is the production of a culture of binary certainty, either the criteria have been met or they have not. The outcomes, or at least, certain selected outcomes, of the service are the subject of apparently precise measurement and contractual agreement. However, in one sense, they tell us little about the detail and context of care delivery:

> 'Target immunisation rates of 95% polio, diphtheria and tetanus by age 18 months; 91% pertussis by 18 months; 93% measles, mumps and rubella by

age two. . . . Evidence that staff resources are targeted in areas where there is a high risk in child protection work; evidence that health service staff have been offered the correct immunisation by the occupational health department; evidence of appropriate staff update in current techniques and emergency procedures . . . and what we do in our monitoring meeting is we provide reports that will demonstrate, for example, the numbers of areas of training, how many staff have been trained and in which specific areas . . . '
(community manager, Sceptical Health Services Trust)

Even the conceptual framework within which nursing care is delivered is also a subject, at least in theory, for formalising and monitoring, although it is difficult to imagine how this might be 'monitored' in a way that actually has any relation to care delivered. But perhaps that is not the point. The point is rather the gesture to formalise even such an abstract and widely questioned notion as a nursing model. Nothing, even (or perhaps, especially) the thinking processes of the nurse must lie outside the range of the formalised, the verifiable, the contractable:

[reads] '. . . . "Nursing care is based upon recognised nursing model."'
(community manager, Sceptical Health Services Trust)

Of particular interest in the interview texts are instances where managers from nursing backgrounds, figures who might be considered nursing 'leaders' within their Trusts work out detailed responses to the problem of the measurability of nursing work. Although often ventured in confident terms, I suggest that these passages can be seen as enacting a struggle between discourses that are irreconcilable, examples of speakers placed in positions where it is almost impossible to achieve and present a unified subjectivity. One such passage shows a nurse executive presenting a discourse that attempts to distance itself from a mainstream view of health care by associating it with 'science', 'men', and 'the medical profession' who play 'the numbers game'. However, as in other passages, such attempts appear to end with attempts to enrol (Callon *et al.* 1986) nurses in a managerial project by recommending that they take up the dominant language and mentality of numerical measurement *in their own interests*:

INTERVIEWER: One of the things that health visitors have said, is it's virtually impossible to demonstrate your effectiveness, this person says you could spend two hours with a client and how can you show that it might have prevented them, you know, being admitted to say casualty, do you think health visitors have got a particular dilemma?

NURSE EXECUTIVE: Yes I do think they have a particular dilemma, because they, I think they have really, yes, because one of the things that happens in health care is that if you do all the stuff that is quantifiable, like the numbers game and number crunching then you definitely can prove something in the view, I have to say it, of men in the medical profession, who think they own science and research . . .

Here the discourse refers to and relies upon nursing's political and philosophical struggle with medicine often identified with 'science' by nurses. Yet there is a distancing too from this 'alternative' discourse in nursing because it is proposed that it is in nurses' interests to be able to 'demonstrate' that they are doing something effective. Managers sometimes, as here, questioned the morality of nurses by suggesting that they hid behind a professional mystique of unquantifiability. In this way they could undercut nurses' own claims to be the supremely moral actors:

' . . . a health visitor must know why they went round and tried to convince the mother to breast feed, and it is not because in fifty years time she will still be on this earth and be able to measure whether that person had coronary heart disease or not, or whether they were in good health, what ever that may be, and what they have got to get used to doing is when they write their care plans, actually give research evidence of why they have actually given that piece of information, 'cause it would certainly make them think. . . . And I think that what they need to be able to do is sit down and clearly think through in their teams how they will review their work and how they will demonstrate what they are doing. . . . Immunisation is a classic one, it is a real number crunchy one which health visitors can get into. In a way they almost don't like doing it, they don't want, I think health visitors have got to make up their minds what it is they want to do . . . '

(nurse executive, Pragmatic Community Health Services)

The speaker proposes a new project for nurses to embark upon. It is a work that managers require in order to demonstrate their own efficient use of public funds and to be seen to be in control of the detail of activity in their organisations, but the unspoken implication is that the survival of certain groups of community nurse depends too upon this 'demonstration'. They have to 'make up their minds', 'sit down' and enter into the project of increasing explicitness and formally rational activity.

'Nobody has got outcome sorted out, nobody has got health gain sorted out . . . the trouble is that health care is so incredibly complex it is very difficult to do that, but I think every nurse in the community, who ever they may be, if you are a district nurse you can measure a wound and you can measure if it is closing up or not and healing, and that is something very quantifiable. Immunisation for health visitors, I'm trying to think of something for school nursing, number of children that have less days of absenteeism from school perhaps, because they have actually dealt with the problem that was affecting their school attendance, there is all sorts of things they can use, less pregnancies . . . '

(nurse executive, Pragmatic Community Health Services)

I would not want to argue that such attempts at 'measurement' are inappropriate on the grounds that they might compromise the personal relationship that nurses might foster with clients, nor argue idealistically that concretising some of nurses' effects would sully the intuitive aspects of their work. Rather it is the attempt at drawing in community nurses to a language, a project, a mentality which effaces certain aspects of their achievements in the effort to meet managerial needs, running the risk that the character of this work becomes changed in unanticipated and perhaps unwanted ways. In the listing of these examples of outcome in the above passage, the complexity of the work done by nurses and health visitors suffers the same reduction or erasure that this manager has been attempting to avoid in her acknowledgement of health care's 'incredible complex[ity]'.

The sceptics

Measurement and recording may have been powerful new tools in the hands of those placed to scrutinise the results and determine relevant action to be taken, but those placed differently in these organisations experienced them as far from empowering. The sceptics were clear about the disadvantages of the recent emphasis on the monitoring and measurement of activity within their Trusts. This group of managers were more likely to use frankly economic terminology, 'earn money', 'throughput' and 'meeting the contracts', not because they were committed to economic rationalism but rather because they distanced themselves from it. The blunter the language they could associate with a managerial project, the stronger the dualism they could form between that and the 'human' values of 'forming relationships' and 'face-to-face contact' that they saw as marginalised by the discourse of rationalism. The following speaker's repeated use of the verb 'get' suggests the pressure of disembodied achievement; the reaching of targets appears to have become an end in itself because of the pressure of being called to 'justify' any shortfall to senior management:

> 'I think we're pressurised quite a lot on the financial side. I think we're pressurised in our daily plan of action if you like, within the trust to earn money when that's, I feel has come to the fore, much more than it had before . . . we've got to get the patient throughput, we've got to get numbers, get the mileage right, we do spend a lot of time looking . . . to try and make sure that we're meeting the contracts that we have. I find it really stressful because on my desk every month comes this [document] done in terms of numbers. I have to go and justify them. . . . Its very stressful. . . . '
> (health visitor manager, Brick-built Hospital Trust)

Other sceptical managers spoke explicitly about how the recording of selective activity lent legitimacy to these acts, while causing others to remain invisible, and about the insensitivity of numerical measurement to the deteriorating economic and social context within which many community nurses were targeting their work. The result of falling activity levels is described in the language of hostility 'we are judged' and 'threatened'. As part of one argument, a manager juxtaposes another piece of recent government terminology, the 'total package of care', against activity level-based contracting:

> 'I think the way that the contracts are based now on activity, activity levels, it doesn't take into account all the sort of total package of care, face to face contact, and, for example, [contacting] St. Michael's, [hospice] . . . and our activity is dropping and we are judged on that. We'd be threatened that we are going to be losing some of our money because of it.'
>
> (local manager, Pragmatic Community Health Services)

Occasionally, managers were openly cynical about the political use made of purportedly objective measures of efficiency and about how such measuring could be manipulated:

> 'I mean, you get all these waiting-list things out but I mean, really, say for casualty, it's when you hit the triage nurse. They don't say how long you sit from then on in, so I think, actually, in a way, the public is slightly conned by all of this. I mean, I think it's a good thing to actually say what you are doing and look at your service in depth, because I think we are accountable, . . . we've got to be accountable, but I think the methods of doing it are a bit of a con to the public, quite honestly.'
>
> (local manager, Pragmatic Community Health Services)

Managers told stories of how there were strong drives for particular kinds of numerical order within their organisations in spite of the fact that in the process, endless contextual knowledge was erased:

> 'Now some time ago, I was asked to draw up a sort of list of priorities and I didn't. I said that the priority as far as I was concerned is that if a patient deteriorates because you don't visit, then that means that they've got to be visited and that it's very difficult to write a list of priorities. . . . However, there is a list now of different priorities: 1, 2, 3 or 4. Ones where you actually must visit, ones which, OK, could be left a day or two or what have you. . . . '
>
> (nurse advisor, Pragmatic Community Health Services)

Nevertheless, as we read further, an authority invested in 'science' is, according to this speaker, inappropriately ascribed to 'rough rules of thumb' with an oppressive result that 'frightens' the speaker and, as we can now see, is characteristically linked to a financial penalty. An impersonality and inflexibility is made to follow from this science of numbers as the authority of personal professional judgement is replaced by a managerial algorithm:

> ' . . . what I'm concerned about is that they [the priorities] are quite broad and OK, do it as a rough guide, but what frightens me is when general management then take them as a scientific proof, you know, and I've heard

someone say "Oh well, you know their priority list is very low; they don't need as many District Nurses as that" . . . it is simplifying something that isn't simple.'

(nurse advisor, Pragmatic Community Health Services)

To summarise, the sceptics described measurement as running against the grain of their own professional judgement which they described as complex and highly contextual and as being the mechanism for an oppressive power over them. Yet at the same time, it appeared to facilitate certain aspects of their subjectivity as they contrasted it with their own identification with the human, the imprecise and the unquantifiable.

THE PHYSICS OF FINANCE

The rationality of finance was generally called upon as a virtually immovable structure giving rise to a law of cause and effect as simple and inescapable as any found in the physical sciences. This way of speaking of the constraints of finance, of the need to 'balance the books', as law-like could effectively erase most traces of political or moral choice, for example government taxation policy, and its ideological basis. This financial awareness was often contrasted with a previous era or previous consciousness when such a law either did not operate or operated in some indirect and far removed way in NHS organisations. Managers often contrasted their own enlightenment to this state of affairs, this unavoidable truth, with the primitive and irrational attitudes of those in their organisations who had not or would not come to this realisation.

Sometimes financial laws were invoked as the foundation upon which evaluations and judgements were based and legitimised. At other times managers discussed financial principles in close proximity to passages discussing rationality in a broader sense. As we shall see, in this proximity, a link was made by managers between financial rationality and any behaviour or approach that merited being taken seriously.

At moments speakers would enact a distancing from the financial imperatives of managing health care. As Swales and Rogers suggest in their study of company mission statements, 'the profit motive can be rhetorically problematic since it can appear to conflict with high "ethical" tone and "human" values . . . ' (Swales and Rogers 1995: 232). The same may be true when describing the financial aspects of providing health care. There may be a certain awkwardness:

'Well, I mean we are being asked to provide services that are efficient and effective, but when we are looking at efficiency, I suppose we are coming into an area of doing the most work, um, doing it as it should be done, but doing it, I suppose for the least amount of – using resources the best way we can.'

(community manager, Sceptical Health Services Trust)

More usually financial acumen was a skill which managers owned up to having with great enthusiasm, sometimes apparently eager to describe themselves and their activities with its terminology. In the following passages, there is a combination of financial language, 'shifting investment', 'rationalising assets' and a language of detached almost gleeful problem-solving, 'really, really interesting', 'looking at' (see p. 107 for a discussion of metaphors of 'looking at'). There is perhaps an implied demystifying and disempowering of medicine involved in the claim and act of applying generalisable business principles:

'The "out of town" contracts [with GP fundholders] are really, really interesting because that's been around looking at skill mix, changing skill mix, shifting investment from straight community nursing to the supporting Physios, OTs. . . . '

(chief executive, Optimist Community Health Trust)

'I don't approach the general management of psychiatric services any differently to the way I approach the community services. You know, we've gone through very much of the same debate about rationalising assets with, for example, our community hospitals that we are now looking at for the acute psychiatric facility, so we use very, very similar approaches, yes.'

(ibid.)

Many managers presented themselves as embracing and facilitating the financial influence of 'market forces' as strengthening the service ethos of the NHS. Such an influence granted managers a new authority over their employees.

'We've lost a couple of small contracts, only small, but because of attitude, no more than attitude. Not because of standards, clinical standards or staff standards but because of attitude . . . our staff will have to come to terms with it more and more. If they don't treat the purchaser and his patients with respect, with dignity, with positive attitude, they'll lose business and we'll wind down the number of staff.'

(chief executive, Sceptical Health Services Trust)

In this passage, the speaker uses the talk of market forces to achieve a rhetorical reversal of nurses' claims for moral supremacy by associating the rhetoric of 'respect, dignity and positive attitude' with the gravitational 'winding down' of staffing levels. It is the 'staff's' ability to deliver a caring service that becomes the dubious moral unknown in this equation. The impersonality of financial forces enables managers to adopt a stance of neutrality, almost noninvolvement, a disingenuous exclusion of the political context of decision-making. However, simultaneously with acknowledging the disembodied existence of such forces, many managers asserted their own potency to act with the flow and force of nature, of an inner logic, an ontology of financial rationality:

' . . . the dentists, have actually got a bit of flab around and can manage to lose a bit of money so actually what we do is we manoeuvre the budget in house, with the agreement of the DHA. Now what we did with the doctors last year was, they were, almost had, well, they had no job to do, Michael. It was just, the fact that GPs had taken over child surveillance, rightly or wrongly, I'm not there to comment on the politics of it, whether its a good idea. It had happened and they just were not fully occupied so we made them redundant and I've done the same thing with the dentists last week. I made six dentists redundant.'

(nurse executive, Pragmatic Community Health Services)

By constituting the financial activities of the Trust as proceeding from a realm of the impersonal, managers could adopt the language of offering their staff autonomy while exercising detailed control themselves:

'My view is now that I should be able to say to the nurses you have this amount of money, and I don't mind how you use it, as long as you follow these types of criteria, focus on these priorities and we expect this quality of work and we expect these hours covered.'

(chief executive, Pragmatic Community Health Services)

Elsewhere, a manager appeals to talk of teamwork between the professional and client, of user empowerment, to, disingenuously in my view, suggest that decision-making and power is exercised at the level of the individual client and health care worker. This conceals financial decisions which have already been made by others. It is achieved through the use of the colloquial metaphors 'bottom line' and 'money in the pot' implying commonplace and unalterable realities. These privilege financial talk over the various and imprecise 'ways that you can talk about needs':

' . . . there's an awful lot of different ways that people express their needs and an awful lot of ways that you can – or an awful lot of ways that you can talk about needs, like felt needs, expressed needs, demands. The bottom line is that there is only so much money in the pot so they [health visitors] and the client have to decide together the best way of managing their care.'

(nurse executive, Pragmatic Community Health Services)

In another passage, a middle manager forged a similar link between patient choice and financial forces. In this case 'thinking about the viability' of her directorate and an ever vigilant concern for 'what our clients need' are linked rhetorically rather than logically. What is clear and enacted in the text is the element of personal pressure and responsibility. What is not so clear is the direct link between financial viability and sensitivity to local health needs. Given that one of the major planks of the government's market reforms was responsiveness to the needs and preferences of the public, it is not surprising that this language is adopted by managers as they (are forced to) take a position towards what is assumed to be the impact of 'market forces'. In the following extract, the first person pronoun is used with activities associated with vulnerability and scrutiny. It is even switched to mid-sentence to emphasise the personal pressure yet the more distant second person is used to describe the element of 'looking at' client need:

> 'I have to spend a lot of time thinking about the viability of the Directorate . . . you've actually got to – I, myself, have to be very clear that there is no guarantee that our service has got jobs for life so all the time you have to be looking at what our clients need. . . . '
>
> (community manager, Sceptical Health Services Trust)

This passage includes what is by far the most frequently occurring metaphor in the interviews, that of 'looking at' as a figure for considering or attempting to understand. At the very least it suggests a certain physical distance or a non-engaging overview or scanning but it also carries echoes of the Enlightenment's spectator subject surveying nature. There are also ideas of dominance and control associated with this conception of knowing because of the way the object of knowledge is equated with what is available to, or present to, or grasped by, the consciousness of the subject (Levinas 1996). This conception reduces the heterogeneity of appearances into whatever is present to the subject and in turn creates the possibility of their control by that subject (Benhabib 1990: 111). We are reminded of Foucault's descriptions of the art of ever more penetrating seeing that he argues was a characteristic of seventeenth- and eighteenth-century European disciplinary societies (an extension to which can be found in the development of computerised and other methods of recording and regulating activity referred to in the interviews). Furthermore, Richard Rorty speaks of Western notions of knowledge as dominated by 'Greek ocular metaphors' (Rorty 1980: 11) and Derrida of Cartesian images of 'natural light' as the light that manifests the truth (Derrida 1982b: 267).

In a similar passage to the one quoted previously (see p. 99), financial consciousness is linked, dubiously perhaps, with improved patient care. A managerial initiative to 'push . . . forward' cost-consciousness and time management practices among field staff is associated with better care through the ambiguously worded suggestion that nurses will 'be able to do more for their patients' within the resource and time constraints that they have:

> ' . . . people are becoming more conscious of the money, and I think that is very important. . . . And people need to start thinking like that because then they will be able to do more for their patients by using their time more effectively, so we are pushing all of that forward.'
>
> (chief executive, Pragmatic Community Health Services)

In the following passage, the financial framework of life in the NHS is described as a foundational reality. The self-conscious bluntness of the language helps to make convincing the marginalising of those who might question it, not only in a health care context but 'in most things'. The move to universalise this 'reality' also acts to support the statement, although there is a characteristic withdrawing from too strong an utterance (perhaps because of the possible conflict with 'human' values alluded to above); money is only 'one of the bottom lines':

> 'We get 12 million pounds from the DHA and they say to us, "that's to provide your total community health service" – that's it. Bonk! . . . I – lets be blunt about it. . . . There's no point in – you would be foolish to ever think that money wasn't one of the bottom lines in most things.'
>
> (nurse executive, Pragmatic Community Health Services)

In the context of this framework, part of the manager's mission in the new NHS is to colonise other workers who might not share the same world view. Again, any view contrary to one in which finance is central is marginalised as foolish. Those who hold to this view are described as not understanding, needing education, seeing things in 'very simple terms', suffering from naive delusions of believing 'there are pots of money' or that 'somebody's going to come and bail them out'. Perhaps in order to reserve a position of overview, this speaker understates her criticism of such naivety and describes it, not as immoral or plain stupid, but as 'interesting'. Nevertheless, the statement claims a final authority in its short unequivocal last phrase:

> '[We need to] educate them [GP fundholders]. We don't keep that a secret. We say that's real. If you want your health visitor to visit people 20 miles away you've got to realise you've got to pay her travel costs. Can you afford it? They don't understand some of those practical nitty-gritty issues. They see it in very simple terms quite often . . . people seem to think there are pots of money, its very interesting that they think if they overspend somebody's going to come and bail them out. But in fact they're not.'
>
> (nurse executive, Pragmatic Community Health Services)

Often managers referred to financial rationality and to a contrast between rational and irrational thinking in such close proximity (within 15 lines of transcript) that the two discourses became associated and mutually supportive in each other's presence. For example, in one passage, part of running 'good services' is described as being able to demonstrate that they are 'cost-effective' so that their value becomes verifiable and explicit. A contrast is then made between the notion of demonstrable value and staff irrationality and fearfulness and one aspect of 'professionalism':

' . . . we have worked very, very hard at getting everybody to work closely with their GP . . . and if we are running good services, more cost-effectively because of the kind of benefits, cost benefits of scale, support, training, and 24 hour cover and things, then we shouldn't be worried about the fact that the GPs are going to have to budget for buying them.

If we think that what we are doing is a good job, then we ought to be able to explain that to people. And if we can't explain that to people, then perhaps we are not doing a good job. There is an issue round in the health service, about what I call professional preciousness, and it is no good saying we are good, because we are good, you have to be able to say we are good because we do this, we do that, and we do the other, and look, if we don't do this that and the other then that happens. I mean GPs come out of school at 18 the same as you and I did, and by and large they are ordinary, sensible reasonable human being[s], there is the odd GP who is really difficult. . . . '

(chief executive, Pragmatic Community Health Services)

'Professional preciousness' is constructed by contrast with a mainstream reason-ableness characteristic of 'ordinary, sensible, reasonable human being[s]', a quality that overrides professional boundaries and is possessed by anyone with moderate intelligence, who came 'out of school at 18'. The discourse explicitly addresses and includes the listener as a subject who shares this reasonableness.

RATIONALITY CONTRASTED WITH VARIOUS FORMS OF IRRATIONALITY

Managers frequently defined and enhanced their own rationality by forming a contrast to their staff's suspicion, traditionalism, impermeability to information, fearfulness, tendency to complain rather than constructively problem-solve and reluctance to plan. In this respect they were everything that staff were not. It could be said that this difficulty, seen from the managers' point of view, characterised relations with care-delivery staff. If staff were unwilling to support management, it was because of a lack of understanding, rather than disagreement, and a sign that managers needed to 'do more work' with these individuals or groups or devise or refine another 'strategy'. For example, one manager spoke about staff's response to the suggestion of the introduction of team formation and changes in skill-mix:

'[When we told] the district nurses about [skill-mix/team formation], some were sceptical because our management changed, "that means they're going to save money and that means it's not going to be as good as it was before", or whatever. Some sort of said "yes", they thought it was a good idea, actually probably a chance for promotion and the vast majority weren't actually interested as long as it didn't affect them directly – and the intention was that it wouldn't.'

(nurse executive, Optimist Community Health Trust)

All of the responses are viewed as examples of different aspects of irrationality; those who are against change are so from prejudice, as the caricature of their (possibly perceptive) reaction suggests, those who are for it are self-interested (hardly an entirely unworthy motive, one would imagine in an organisation where managers wish to shake off negativity) and the vast majority are indifferent to change that does not impinge on them; again their indifference suggests that they are far from fully participative, motivated workers. However, the very indifference of staff has been taken into account by management when introducing sensitive measures like these skill-mix changes – 'the intention was that [the change] wouldn't [affect them]'. As a result of this change, and as a ratification of the intrinsic sense behind it, 'a natural flow down, natural hierarchy within the team' appeared. In a sense, this manager describes his activity as allowing what is natural to emerge.

A key project among most managers was to change fundamental attitudes of their workforce. The difference between what could be called the caring orientation of qualified nurses and a newer managerial role was often described in terms of the difference between irrationality and systematic and intelligent planning: 'we had to get them away from the "I am the District Nurse and I must do everything for all my patients"' (nurse executive, Optimist Community Health Trust). Nurses were even described with the imagery of mental illness. Quintessentially irrational, nurses could react with a 'meganeurosis' about skill-mix. Senior doctors were seen to exhibit the same irrationality by 'shouting': ' . . . consultants in particular . . . shouting "more of this, more of that." Somebody has to stand back and say "What gives us the most health gain?"' (chief executive, Sceptical Health Services Trust). Metaphors privileging 'standing back', 'sitting down', 'looking' abounded in this discourse, emphasising physical distance and mental activity.

Some saw the achievement of this as an aspect of advancing professional consciousness:

'I think whereas every nurse will have a care plan in her head perhaps for the patients, it has to be better to actually have to be explicit about the care plan and if we're going to look at how effective we're being, we must be able to evaluate the care that is being given and we are encouraging our staff to become reflective practitioners. They must be able to evaluate their work and decide whether that has in fact been the most effective way of treating that patient.'

(community manager, Sceptical Health Services Trust)

Another nurse executive constructed an image of nurses' irrationality. She described two simultaneous yet contradictory responses from nurses faced with apparently unmeetable need among their patients. Their very incompatibility reinforces her point about nurses' irrationality. The first response is frenetic, unreflective activity *par excellence*: Nurses may:

> ' . . . go around like headless chickens the whole time, trying to fulfil so many roles and be everything to everybody, but I think that is the nature of nursing that that is the way that they feel they ought to behave.'
> (nurse executive, Pragmatic Community Health Services)

The second response she identified was more subtle but equally unreflective. It was an unconscious rationing or covert priority setting:

> 'All the research shows that they are the people who have been rationing for years and years at the front line. Nurses that work at the coal face have been doing it. They probably would find it quite interesting if people pointed out to them how they decided on their caseloads, who was going to be seen and in what order and why and how.'
> (ibid.)

The problem with both these responses, according to this nurse executive, was their lack of reflection; they are not consciously adopted approaches that may lead either to effective working, reduced stress or a well-articulated professional strategy. More importantly, perhaps, they are not available for scrutiny and control because of their informal nature. It was here that this nurse executive felt there was an appropriate area for professional 'leadership'. In the face of health and social need that she acknowledges as 'infinite', management:

> ' . . . actually have to be able to say very clearly to nurses what it is we expect of them within their current job, or within the resources they have, so that they don't go around like headless chickens . . . and I suppose that is part of changing the culture of nursing slightly.'
> (ibid.)

Changing the culture of nursing, whether slightly or fundamentally, would involve, she believed, developing a professional who can articulate her rationales for activity, objectives, outcomes as well as unmet need. A more collected, reflective practitioner (the metaphor of nurses 'sitting down' was repeated) would be more confident and articulate, to the benefit of the profession and more monitorable by the organisation:

> 'I think that health visitors nevertheless can't hide behind "it is too difficult to prove what we are doing", and I think it is time that they sat down and thought very clearly. . . . '
> (ibid.)

Here 'hiding' undercuts any moral stance that may be taken by professionals by introducing a suggestion of lack of intellectual and moral nerve.

Although the language of the three nurse executives involved in this study differed, their diagnoses of nursing's ills and their prescriptions were similar; that nursing must become a more rationally focused activity. One nurse executive's unease with the term 'caring' as a description of nursing, in this light, was significant, along with her wish to reconstitute nursing in terms of its complexity:

> 'I really hate the word "care", but I don't know what other word to use really, 'cause it sort of smacks of something that isn't quite what nursing really is about . . . it makes it sound like some rather shilly-shally job that anybody could do. . . . when it is one of the most complex jobs that any human being does in this world.'
>
> (nurse executive, Pragmatic Community Health Services)

Here again, it is possible to detect vestiges of a previous discourse relating to nursing as a moral calling, suggested subtly by the grand rhetoric of 'any human being . . . in the world'. Yet in this ambiguous statement 'caring', the traditional watchword of the nursing profession is excluded as parasitic upon the more valuable notion of complexity.

Postmodernism alerts us to the language and technologies of power that are available within modernity to coercive institutions of various kinds. In this chapter, I have argued that managers presented themselves within a context of a rationality that both legitimised their own discourse and actions, and subjugated the knowledge of other groups. Describing their actions as rational or flowing from reason erases their own interested position and associates their decisions with the authority of some external given. In the next chapter we will go on to examine some of the main subjects and objects of managerial discourse along with their modernist constructions of autonomy and tradition.

7 The interviews part II: subjects and objects, autonomy and tradition

SUBJECTS AND OBJECTS

A useful way to begin an analysis of discourse is to identify its subjects and objects (Parker 1992). I have already discussed how discourses have been seen as 'practices that systematically form the objects of which they speak' (Foucault 1972: 49) and how discourse can give rise to subjects who listen to, read, speak or write the texts discourses inhabit. In addition, I have also explored a little of how 'a discourse makes available a space for particular types of self to step in' (Parker 1992: 9). We might call these spaces subject positions.

In this chapter I want to explore a number of such subject positions which speakers involved in this research appeared to adopt, as well as a range of 'objects' created by their discourse. Where it is useful, I have separated a mainstream managerial approach from how the sceptics positioned themselves towards various subject positions or objects of discourse. (See Chapter 5, p. 88 for an explanation of managerial 'sceptics').

Subject positions

Acting in the public interest

A central aim of the NHS reforms and of a subsequent key government document, the *Patient's Charter* (Department of Health 1991), was to increase the service's responsiveness to its clients. The *Charter*, which was quickly followed by a number of local and organisational 'charters' defined, for example, acceptable and unacceptable waiting times and standards for the provision of information to clients and patients. I have already summarised arguments that with this move the government could achieve three things: they could constitute themselves and their policies as caring, signal a move away from a left-wing impersonal state planning model to a more consumerist model and steal the high ground from the professions whose position has traditionally rested upon a claim that they act in the public's interest (Pollitt 1993). Nevertheless, it would be inaccurate to suggest that these initiatives amounted to little more than a cynical exercise in public relations. It seems likely that the charter movement focused the attention of at least some of those involved in health care on issues of concern to its users such as waiting lists and waiting times.

At some stage during the interviews most managers (as well as the nursing workforce in their own comments) offered this concern as a foundation for their actions. 'Acting in the public interest' was a versatile position; it could be adopted to support the arguments and aspirations of community trusts who wished to win contracts for procedures from hospital rivals and ' . . . break this hospital domination. . . . Most people don't want to be in hospital' (chief executive, Pragmatic Community Health Services); it could be used to justify financial control: ' . . . all this public money we're spending and you and I are taxpayers and we [i.e. NHS employees] should be more accountable' (nurse executive, Sceptical Health Services Trust); to justify moves to blur traditional demarcations between professional roles: 'Mr Jones out there with multiple sclerosis could do with patient focused care – one professional who did everything. Now, we can do that with our support worker staff . . . ' (chief executive, Pragmatic Community Health Services); and to issue sideswipes at the professions:

> 'In my view [the business ethos] is there to make us all aware of the importance of treating people as they should be treated and not merely in the clinical sense.'
>
> (chief executive, Sceptical Health Services Trust)

This was a subject position that speakers could take up and simultaneously further arguments in support of their interests, and be seen to be acting in harmony with government policy.

During the course of the interviews, it was sometimes possible to suspect that rhetoric and the reality of practice became confused within the arguments of some managers:

> 'Everything is done with the client's needs in perspective first, and the professional needs following up the rear, rather than worrying about what the professionals want and then deciding what the clients can have as a result, which I think has tended to happen in the past.'
>
> (nurse executive, Pragmatic Community Health Services)

At a point of unprecedented public financial stringency, when, due to pressure of work, some community nurses in the Trusts under study were set a 'core function', that is, a minimal range of interventions, the claim that 'everything is done with the client's need' first, seems disingenuous. It is unconvincing that such a thorough break with the past has been achieved. This passage enacts, I suggest, the persuasive and self-persuasive power of rhetoric.

At about the time of the third-year interviews, there had been considerable publicity about government claims that waiting lists for various hospital procedures had shortened as a result of its reforms. Its *Patient's Charter* had attempted to set explicit waiting targets. One of the 'sceptics' took up the government's own rhetoric and used it, albeit with attempts to soften the critical edge of her words, to challenge the sincerity of its claims. Though the content of her comment is less comfortable than the previous speaker's because of its direct challenge to government rhetoric, her position is clearly orientated to the public interest:

'... you get all these waiting list things out but I mean, really, say for casualty, it's when you hit the triage nurse [a nurse whose job is to sort out the serious from the less urgent cases]. They don't say how long you sit from then on in, so I think, actually, in a way, the public is slightly conned by all of this.'

(local manager, Pragmatic Community Health Services)

The words of the following speaker offer a striking example of the struggle for dominance between the new NHS rhetoric of consumer-centredness that we saw in the first comment and a residual discourse that involves talk of a protective attitude towards staff, perhaps the sort of 'nannying' that many managers appeared keen to distance themselves from. The following example of what can be described as a multiple subject position, i.e. the simultaneous striking of positions that are logically incompatible, was discussed in Chapter 3. The passage features a repeated process of readjustment of meaning; first an assertion of the staff's vulnerability, then a more formal statement of patient priority and finally a re-emergence of a sense of responsibility towards the workforce:

'... there's a lot of concern, I mean it's a big responsibility with the numbers of staff that we've got and people dependent on their professions [i.e. livelihoods] and not only [?]this, first and foremost always comes our patients and clients of our service but next very close after that comes our staff and that actually is an even greater responsibility lying on my shoulders.'

(community manager, Sceptical Health Services Trust)

This subject position was adopted, therefore, with different degrees of whole-heartedness – as a space from which to promote organisational ambitions; as a moral standpoint from which to question the government's intention, or, in a more troubled and contradictory way, as a position in which nurses' insecure employment competes with a patient-centred rhetoric. It is this last marginal stance that alerts us to the transitional and incomplete dominance of managerial rationality.

Visionary

Some speakers adopted a language of visionary or charismatic leadership characteristic of much management writing of the 1970s and 1980s (Peters and Waterman 1982) and a style of leadership that has been associated with workforce manipulation through the reconstitution of organisational realities (Rafferty 1993b). This subject position featured reflective comments about leadership, couched in derivative language. In fact, the very unoriginality of the language gives it its associative and almost iconic power: 'I'm very conscious now that I am a leader of an organisation. I certainly believe that one's got to lead from the front and that senior managers must take the initiative . . . I've got to keep the organisation moving forward, developing. . . . A static organisation is a dying organisation' (chief executive, Optimist Community Health Trust), 'I'm more part of this organisation and this organisation is part of me' (nurse executive, Optimist Community Health Trust), 'I'm sort of one of life's eternal optimists that says 'make it work the other way. Make it work strategically. You've got to take control of the process and make sure it happens and . . . galvanise [people] . . . let's be dynamic' (nurse executive, Pragmatic Community Health Services). The position was also characterised by references to new opportunities made available, if not by the reforms themselves, by the energising new thinking that they brought: 'I think becoming a first wave Trust, you are very aware that you are on a sort of leading edge of organisational development' (chief executive, Optimist Community Health Trust). Talk of shaping organisational culture emphasised the managers' sense of potency with suggestions of the religious language of genesis: 'We had the opportunity to start a culture . . . we have an opportunity to make things happen for the first time. . . . Culture is a state of mind. Its what you believe you can do' (nurse executive, Optimist Community Health Trust). The following speaker explicitly, and unusually for the managers, drew upon 'theory' to lend legitimacy to an explanation for staff's resistance to managerial initiatives:

> 'The whole management of change stuff, would be, if you read the theory on this, talks about how people often resist change, because they feel that a change is implicitly saying that what they have been doing so far is bad. And you have to help people see that that is not true, what they were doing before is really good, but now the world is changing, there are new things that we can do, new ways of doing it and being good means doing it differently now.'
>
> (chief executive, Pragmatic Community Health Services)

This passage is notable for two major persuasive moves. First, is the suggestion of altruism and facilitation suggested by talk of 'help[ing] people see', i.e. spreading a particular vision which masks a persuasive project. The second is the language of possibility and freedom used to constitute the new world 'there are new things that we can do, new ways of doing it'. This excludes any mention of constraint or compromise within which both managers and field staff are obliged to operate.

Some managers spoke of 'a vision' for community nursing which involved either its participation in health care activities previously undertaken in hospitals or a belief in the emergence of a new kind of nurse:

'All the time the role of nurses is growing and the impact of nursing upon the health service, if channelled appropriately, is THE most significant factor of all. There are more of us, we are more articulate, the Project 2000 folks that are coming out now, what a powerful weapon that is. You know, highly qualified and lots of them, free, challenging, articulate people who are not being trained to be a bed pan emptier which is great.'

(nurse executive, Optimist Community Health Trust; original emphasis)

The rising note of professional warfare and triumphalism enacted by the first phrases of the passage is brought into strong contrast to the 'bed pan emptier' with its associations of the socially stigmatised activities that some have seen as an explanation for aspects of nursing's invisibility and low status (Lawler 1991). This, and other passages, perform a reconstitution of nursing work as a technical challenge and marginalise some of its so-called menial aspects.

No sceptics adopted this kind of 'visionary' language nor did managers from Sceptical Health Services Trust which was characterised more by the language of problem-solving and remedial activity.

Manager as therapist

Perhaps because of the influence of human resources management (Pollitt 1991), of talk of managers as creators of culture, or as facilitators and nurturers of their staff's abilities (Peters and Waterman 1982), some managers spoke of their strategies as having a beneficial impact on their staff's well-being. This often appeared to involve leading staff where they would not naturally want to go, curbing or shaping their desires, in their own interests. At other times, the therapy in the form of 'showing staff that you value them' took a more overt form:

'We've recently fixed a travel scholarship and that's £1,000 and that's new and the successful candidate is going to San Antonio in Texas for a couple of weeks to study rehabilitation of the elderly. . . . We've introduced our staff recognition scheme which we have made, what we call, distinguished service awards to five staff . . . who were nominated by their colleagues – not by the managers – for exemplifying what we would expect a good employee to be, the people who stay late, arrive early, don't have any time off sick, are happy about their work all the time and, as I said, these are nominated by their colleagues. . . . The Board decided that we would honour one specifically with a particular award as being with the Trust's Distinguished Service Award.'

(nurse executive, Optimist Community Health Trust)

Managers' attempts to shape the culture of the organisations they manage are not always successful because staff who may well inhabit a number of other 'cultures' may show resistance (Drife and Johnston 1995). The speaker quoted above expressed surprise and frustration that staff were reluctant to apply for these awards and could not agree about the design of new uniforms that the board had decided they should wear: 'I've 90-odd district nurses and I've 90-odd answers to what they wanted to wear. I sort of said, "It's really boring, what do you want?" . . . not even the good things people will recognise'. The priorities driving the Distinguished Service Award described above appear to be of such a managerial focus ('the people who stay late, arrive early, don't have any time off sick, are happy about their work all the time') that it is hard to imagine that any worker would put themselves forward for nomination yet they are emphatically presented as driven by the staff.

Another aspect of staff development involved a process that resembles 'coming of age' rituals found within many cultures:

> ' . . . at the end of April, we're taking a group of 10–12 folks away for three days to actually work with them on identifying what their skills, abilities are, what their potential is and hopefully from that group of 12, we will select two, maybe three, folks who have management potential. It's not a pass or fail thing – the others will be – well, perhaps you're a personnel manager, perhaps you're a teacher, perhaps you're a clinician and each person will get a personal development plan which we'll work out with them and then we will mentor them appropriately to achieve their career goal.'
>
> (nurse executive, Optimist Community Health Trust)

This project, like the ones described earlier (see p. 117), involves aligning the personal development of individuals, or at least a particular view of this, with an organisational goal. In the role of therapist, managers, it can be argued, are claiming an almost total power over their employees to the extent that they can gaze into their personal potential and as a result of what they see there, give them new names, 'perhaps you're a personnel manager, perhaps you're a teacher, perhaps you're a clinician'. The preceding two passages are characterised by persistent use of the first person plural, an emphasising and reinforcement, perhaps, of a position characterised by potency, initiative and oligarchy.

The aim of much management activity, including 'management by walking about', road shows, newsletters as well as the schemes just described, was to engender among staff 'a feeling of belonging to a corporate organisation' (chief executive, Optimist Community Health Trust). This was mentioned repeatedly. Again, its ultimate aim appeared to be to harness the personal feelings of individual workers to the organisation's performance:

> '[Such initiatives are] about corporate image, corporate identity, corporate ownership and if you can find a way of making staff feel they belong even more, they're even more of a part of their organisation and even more proud of it. I think that's good for the staff, good for the organisation and good for the people who are being treated.'
>
> (chief executive, Sceptical Health Services Trust)

Sometimes, shaping the consciousness of workers involves giving carefully controlled messages of a less palatable kind:

> ' . . . informing them about certain other issues but hopefully not letting it overwhelm them so that the messages have been quality, standards, look at – carefully appraise what you are doing with your work, why you are doing it the best way, how are we making the best use of all grades . . . There has been a sort of deliberate policy that we shouldn't get people worried before they had to be worried, doesn't mean that we want to sort of nanny them.'
> (community manager, Sceptical Health Services Trust)

Such economically driven urgings to continually examine work practices form almost a parody of the picture of the 'reflective practitioner' described by Schön (1983) and taken up enthusiastically by many nurses. Part of 'making the best use of all grades' involved all the participating Trusts in moves to change the emphasis of the role of the G grade district nursing sister away from care delivery to a more supervisory role. The metaphor of 'nannying' in the passage above was used by some managers and a few nurses. It has also notably been used as a description of what some have seen as a dependence encouraged by welfare provision. The sexist basis of the image and its privileging of independence have been commented on by Davies (1995).

Many managers were aware of the difficulty of instituting changes in patterns of skill-mix and the change of mentality among their staff that they felt was necessary for the successful functioning of these new arrangements. The strategy they adopted towards this tended to be described in therapeutic language: ' . . . we try to support them [nursing staff] through that and give them the skills that they needed to make that change' (community manager, Sceptical Health Services Trust), ' . . . help people see that the world is changing', 'changes are not things to be frightened of, changes are things to kind of use as opportunities. There is no such thing as a problem, only lots of challenges' (chief executive, Pragmatic Community Health Services). Other managerial initiatives, such as the introduction of performance-related pay, which are arguably responses to financial imperatives were also described in therapeutic language:

> 'If you have a true and proper skill-mix as opposed to a cost cutting exercise, you actually end up with people who are happier because they are doing jobs that use their skills rather than jobs that are actually a bit boring.'
> (chief executive, Pragmatic Community Health Services)

In this quotation, the chief executive rhetorically distances herself and her activities from '[im]proper' skill-mix by describing her approach as the authentic 'real thing'. As none of the nurses in this study spoke of so-called basic care as 'boring' and appeared to be orientated towards the personal encounter of caring, it is possible that this manager has misunderstood the motivation of many nurses. Her view, however, is consistent with those of the nurse executives who, in their understanding of their nursing workforce, appeared to correlate sense of reward with technical complexity. Nevertheless, what is important about this passage is the claim that skill-mix changes can have a therapeutic effect for staff.

The sceptics did not appear to adopt this position.

Revolutionary

Many, if not all speakers described themselves as involved in a unique period in the history of the NHS. It was a unique moment to challenge the authority of various immovable structures and positions. The reforms enabled local employers to determine their own rates of pay and to depart from nationally agreed levels set down by the Whitley Councils that were established in 1948 along with the National Health Service (Hart 1994). One speaker described his Trust's initiatives set against the traditional-mindedness and poor imagination of his nursing workforce. His ironic religious imagery parodies this traditionalism: 'We were challenging the fabric of what [nurses] understood, we were challenging Whitley. Well, Whitley was handed down with Moses' (nurse executive, Optimist Community Health Trust). None of the managers included in this analysis had a medical background therefore, perhaps not surprisingly, they saw themselves as challengers of what they saw as a long-standing medical dominance of health services. One chief executive asked, archly, and perhaps significantly, in the same interview that she had spoken of difficult relationships with new consultant psychiatrists employed within the Trust, whether the government was right to stipulate the involvement of consultant medical staff in general management. She argued that doctors often had no management training and could only fulfil such a role to the detriment of their medical responsibilities. In another Trust, the fact that its managers had made a number of community physicians redundant was offered as unmistakeable proof that they had sufficient power and nerve to tackle doctors (although it could be argued that part-time community physicians hardly represent the main core of medical dominance):

> 'We tackle the fact the doctors no longer had any work to do. . . . People might not like it but we do but there's a lot of units who will not address those issues and won't tackle the consultant, won't ask them why one of them's got their hernia in bed for four hours and one of them's got him in bed for four weeks.'
>
> (nurse executive, Pragmatic Community Health Services)

Managers in the Community Trusts that participated spoke of themselves as well placed to challenge 'this hospital domination that we have in this country' (chief executive, Pragmatic Community Health Services) and the traditional power brokers who were identified with hospital institutions:

> 'England is terribly conservative, with a little c, about ever trying anything different and we needed something that broke the power of the traditional

power holders who were the acute usually teaching hospitals and the consultants within them.'

(ibid.)

Managers with a nursing background could also call on this revolutionary position as part of their challenge to medical dominance:

'I think in 10 years time, nurses will be providing quite a lot of the care that doctors currently provide. In fact I'm not sure quite what doctors are going to do, but you know that's their problem, *they're* going to have to worry about that.'

(nurse executive, Pragmatic Community Health Services; original emphasis)

However, it was above all tradition of almost any kind that was being, at least verbally, assaulted. In many passages where the professions were discussed, traditionalism was constituted as entrenchment and reaction. Nursing was also seen to have its fair share of traditions and traditionalists. I will examine the 'traditional nurse' as an object of discourse later. One nurse executive described her task, with characteristically strong language, as being to 'break some of the traditional ways of working' (nurse executive, Sceptical Health Services Trust), and one chief executive talked about ' . . . undoing years of bad habits. I think one or two of the old school people find it quite tough' (chief executive, Pragmatic Community Health Services).

There were other ways in which managers spoke of themselves as revolutionary. For most, the reforms meant that intention and planning were now matched by cash, perhaps borrowed under new financial arrangements. This, some said, set them apart from any of their NHS predecessors, as men and women of action grounded in the reality of observable fact as opposed to the erstwhile idealists: ' . . . *we* can point to the facts. Now, before, we could point to ideals' (nurse executive, Optimist Community Health Trust; original emphasis). However, for some, the reforms were above all described as ushering in a new way of thinking or at least of talking, rather than additional finance: ' . . . getting people to realise that what we used to do is not acceptable, accepting poor standards, you don't have to, you can't say "Well, we haven't got the staff or the money", I don't believe them' (chief executive, Sceptical Health Services Trust). This characterising within the Sceptical Health Services Trust of the past as not acceptable, contrasts with the more carefully placed comment of a previous speaker who emphasised change as not disqualifying previous approaches (chief executive, Pragmatic Community Health Services). This contrast is indicative of the overall differences in management vocabularies between these two organisations; in Sceptical Health Services Trust there was more remedial and less charismatic language.

Risk-taker

This subject position combines something of an entrepreneurial discourse with the learning-by-making-mistakes, or the 'learning organisation' advocated by some management writers (Jones and Hendry 1992). It was directly referred to by virtually every senior manager. 'It has meant making some investment at risk without being sure that we were going to have the revenue to support it' (chief executive, Optimist Community Health Trust). 'We changed from a really traditional structure to one where its alright to make a mistake. In actual fact, if we don't make a mistake, how will we learn and develop and grow?' (nurse executive, Optimist Community Health Trust) Risk-takers contrasted their mentality with a previous one in their organisations where, they suggested, hierarchy, ingrained tradition, professional-centredness and the bureaucracy of central planning removed any chance of risk-taking. Many speakers said that because of this long cultural history, they urgently needed to influence their nursing workforce. Risk-taking was conjured up as desirable with a range of evocative positive attributes and metaphors: 'It is all about being fluid, and enabling and judging and balancing rather than rigid and clear and direct and going into – in *that* direction' (chief executive, Pragmatic Community Health Services; original emphasis).

Transparent

Many speakers described themselves in terms of openness, democracy, a lack of hidden motivation and eagerness to communicate frankly and frequently with staff and to be open to their comments and suggestions. This involved setting up structures with names that emphasised these transparent qualities, 'management by walking about', 'road shows', 'state of the nation speeches' 'team briefing', and 'cascading' information, but also a certain availability, an 'open door policy', a closing of 'the gap between top and bottom' of the employment hierarchy. Their image of leadership was participative even though at other times it had been more concerned with influencing the consciousness and action of staff:

> 'So the more information people have about what's happening, the background and so on, the more they can understand decisions that are being made and the more it allows them to participate in those decisions and to give their thoughts and views. So we want communication to be upwards, almost more than it is downwards.'
> (community manager, Sceptical Health Services Trust)

'Openness' was contrasted with the autocratic management practised either elsewhere in neighbouring organisations or by previous regimes in the same place – 'nobody blew their nose with out asking permission' (chief executive, Pragmatic Community Health Services) yet there was the suggestion that sensitivity to staff, or information giving worked as a way of increasing the effectiveness of managerial decisions by the use of techniques that made them less likely to encounter opposition. One example would be skill-mix changes, a management-driven initiative which was arrived at, in one Trust, through a series of meetings with staff, natural wastage and the acceptance of 'early retirements'. This careful approach was contrasted by managers with the nationally notorious approaches adopted in other areas of the country:

> 'Certainly I didn't go out and say "We've done a skills review, we know it's right and therefore it must happen and if there are casualties, well, that's the way it is."'
>
> (nurse executive, Optimist Community Health Trust)

Paradoxically, perhaps, information-giving was seen to add to the, at times paternalistic, authority of management:

> 'Through communication, accurate communication and giving people that kind of accurate, honest inflow, hopefully confidence will come in management that we know what we're doing, you can trust us, you can rely on us, we'll hopefully come up with the goods on your behalf and your future is as safe as it can be in our hands.'
>
> (nurse executive, Optimist Community Health Trust)

And also to be a part of that authority, as in negotiations over pay with union representatives:

> '[We were] quite happy to negotiate with them [the unions] but at the end of the day we would make the decision and they knew that because that's what we've done and that we wanted to be open with them too, that we didn't have any secrets through that process.'
>
> (nurse executive, Optimist Community Health Trust)

Professional

This subject position, along with that of 'acting in the public interest' was one of only two adopted by the 'sceptics'. I considered that a speaker was adopting this position in passages where they identified their interests or values with that of a particular professional group – in this case nursing. This position did not appear to be available to managers from administrative backgrounds. Unlike most of the other subject positions, this one was usually adopted quite self-consciously. Sometimes, for the nurse executives, moving into this position involved a significant textual shift of perspective, signalled by metaphors such as 'putting a nursing hat on . . . ' (nurse executive, Optimist Community Health Trust). For the 'sceptics' this position was no less self-conscious but a far more integrated part of their subjectivity. For all speakers, the professional position tended to be called upon in order to take a stance against some other outside and possibly threatening group, for example general practitioners or general managers:

> 'What would concern me is if I lost all my district nurses to fundholding GPs, I have great concerns about that from a professional perspective, it's not because my Trust will fall apart if we lost them because it wouldn't, but from a professional perspective, putting a nursing hat on, I have great concerns about that.'
>
> (nurse executive, Optimist Community Health Trust)

Occasionally, when the nurse executives spoke with 'a nursing hat on', they revealed such ambitions for their profession that it was hard to see how these could be reconciled with their corporate responsibilities. It was almost as if there were vestiges of an older or contradictory discourse at work in the texts:

> ' . . . what we could see is the eclipse of nursing as "the senior profession". If we are not promoting nursing and what nursing means, then nursing will become – nurses will become the handmaiden of all the other professions doing the very fundamental care whereas the more intellectually stimulating, more rewarding aspects of caring will be taken over by someone else.'
>
> (nurse executive, Optimist Community Health Trust)

> 'I suppose because of my professional nursing background it is about really seeing nurses come to the forefront and show what their expertise is, and being far more autonomous in the way that they practice.'
>
> (nurse executive, Pragmatic Community Health Services)

The first quotation reveals a particular image of nursing professionalisation. While the term 'handmaiden' has been widely used in nursing literature, usually as a description of the profession's worst possible relationship to medicine, this nurse executive, like managers from administrative backgrounds, identifies the most 'rewarding' nursing work with what is 'intellectually stimulating'. For him, it seems, to be left with the 'very fundamental' care would be a shameful situation for nursing which would not enhance its status. The second comment takes up nursing's characteristically professional concern for autonomy. Again, it forces us to question the place for discourses of autonomy alongside discourses of 'the corporate player'.

The sceptics appealed to professionalism far more frequently than the mainstream managers and it appeared to be a central point of their subjectivity from which the activities and constraints of other groups were evaluated. 'The thinking time that we can bring to actual professional development has often gone into number crunching' (health visitors, Brick-built Hospital Trust). The managers with health visiting backgrounds created a picture of 'professional development' as entirely opaque to those outside the profession such as general practitioners or those responsible for setting contracts in the new NHS:

'As a group of professionals we're looking at the professional way forward. Do you know what I mean? As a professional group and yet they're being asked to integrate into a team which is – that's right as well – and I know certainly from Region or the [Health] Commission, they actually can't understand why health visitors as a profession . . . can't get their support from within the team. "Why can't all these nurses and health visitors get their support from within the team? Why do they have to go out to this other person?" They – its about professional developments and some of them don't want to acknowledge its there.'

(health visitors, Brick-built Hospital Trust)

At other times their professional discourse, along with that of other sceptics, was strikingly similar to less sceptical managers, involving demonstrably rational and sometimes economically implicated procedures. It seemed as if even the sceptics had incorporated, or had little alternative but to incorporate, such elements into the way they spoke about professional behaviour:

' . . . like, Project 2000 based, questioning, objectives led, needs led, assessment, evaluation . . . and I think we're [?somewhere] down the line as a profession, actually going towards that. So we've gone away from the rote, "this must be done at 4, 6 and 9" or whatever, to "does this need to be done for this patient and if so, why?" And to me that's wonderful.'

(health visitors, Brick-built Hospital Trust)

'I think you need to look very critically at what you are doing and to prioritise and think "is the right person doing this?"'

(nurse advisor, Pragmatic Community Health Services)

A range of objects

Perhaps the central feature of any discourse is that it creates objects. This research analyses five prominent objects created by the discourse of managers: the modern world, the good worker, the traditional nurse, dead wood and stress.

The modern world

'The modern world' was frequently cited by managers as the context and justification for their actions. At times some were almost breathlessly excited by this object while the sceptics tended to refer to a similar object with regret or reluctance.

In the discourse of many speakers, the modern world was heralded by new technology, new language, general management, cash-consciousness, markets, sophistication and by 'constant change' (nurse executive, Pragmatic Community Health Services) which left the slow-footed quickly out of date.

In the first year of the study, one manager uttered a litany to modern technology:

> ' – but I mean computers, "Excel Care", the nursing system in [name] Hospital is computer based, "Florence" is a computer based system. Computers are here, wherever we look. A lot of clinical audit work is done on computers, the guys down in the finance department have got computers, my information department has got computers, well of course they have, but so have the nurses. The little gadget I play with, [picks up Psion organiser] that's a computer too and that's just got an electric Filofax on it. There's all sorts of things.'
>
> (nurse executive, Optimist Community Health Trust)

And to the market place, market behaviour and market language:

> 'We're into 1992 and Europe is happening on April 1st – I don't quite know what that means, but anyway – so we have to gear ourselves up a little bit more to compete. There is a market place. I think people are worried by language like that; "a competitive edge", "competing in the market place", and "customers" – we've never talked of any of that stuff before. I actually think we are more efficient an organisation because we've addressed those kinds of issues . . . but that's a bit disconcerting if you've been a district nurse for a long time and suddenly this guy comes along and starts talking about computer systems and programmes and stuff like that.'
>
> (nurse executive, Optimist Community Health Trust)

Part of the definition and a sign of the dynamism of the modern world appears to be the fact that it leaves certain individuals puzzled and worried. Perhaps the conflict between the old and the new worlds is, in some respects, gendered and age-determined, pictured as the confrontation between the mature district nurse and the 'guy' who 'suddenly' appears uttering computer-speak. Along with the well-established district nurse, other victims can be found among the consultant psychiatrists mentioned by another manager who are 'struggling to find a role in the new scheme of things' (chief executive, Optimist Community Health Trust), those who were 'forever harping back to the good old days' (chief executive, Sceptical Health Services Trust) or those clinicians who were 'often trained by people who are out of date with what's going on in the real world' (chief executive, Pragmatic Community Health Services). Those nurses who are not left behind were dubbed by one chief executive, 'technocrats'. She described what she observed as a growing differentiation among her Trust's nurses between traditionalists and others who had turned their backs on a traditional unprofessional mentality and became, it seems, rhetoricians:

> 'Some people say, "The sum of the parts is greater than the whole, what can we do together to actually deliver this agenda? What tools do

we need? How do we utilise these tools? How can we influence general management?" Those people I see more as the technocrats.'

(chief executive, Optimist Community Health Trust)

In a characteristically 'modern' gesture, the shape of this new world was not simply some contingent state of affairs (although it was sometimes figured as that) but was, according to many speakers, part of an ongoing force of historical necessity and increasing complexity:

'We needed people to think about how they were spending their money, to think about more modern and sophisticated ways of doing things.'

(chief executive, Pragmatic Community Health Services)

The sceptics also spoke of a modern world. It appeared to be such a powerful construction that they were forced to describe themselves in relation to it, a relation that was often uncomfortable. Triumphalism and excitement tended to be absent, replaced, as in the following passage, with a jarring series of metaphors that each suggest an element of constraint.

'It's no good digging your head in the sand, you've got to see how nursing is going and make sure that the staff here are on the right road, and they can't be back in Doomsday, you know; we're in 1994 and we've got to make sure that they understand the structure as it were and move with it otherwise we'd all be left behind.'

(nurse advisor, Pragmatic Community Health Services)

Another sceptic told of a recent experience as a hospital patient:

' . . . looking at [it from] my probably old-fashioned view, there wasn't anybody there. For example, somebody would ring a bell and the nurse would shout at the entrance to the ward "Who's ringing? What do you want?" in a loud voice, and someone would have to say "I want a bedpan actually." See what I mean? And I just thought, gosh, is this the modern acceptable way of doing things and perhaps I'm old-fashioned? So I've seen it. . . . '

(local manager, Pragmatic Community Health Services)

She adopts a stance of being 'old-fashioned' in order to ask whether insensitive care is 'acceptable' because it is 'modern' and in this way extends her criticism to the whole NHS. By describing herself as 'old-fashioned', she sets herself apart from both poor standards of care and a 'modern' NHS. Her view of today's health care service appeals to a popular view of the modern world as a place that functions efficiently but which has lost touch with human values. This is a view which the champions of the changes were at pains to distance themselves from.

The good worker

When managers spoke about the 'good worker' it generally had the effect of bridging a gap between themselves and the body of the workforce because it suggested that they were working from a common value base even though one characteristic of the good worker was to be 'challenging' of management. The good worker had a number of characteristics: he or she had taken on an organisation-wide perspective in place of a previous powerful professional tribalism which it had been the task of general management to challenge:

> ' . . . some of them, are starting to embrace . . . the general management agenda and are starting to recognise that the best way they can influence that agenda is by getting involved.'
>
> (chief executive, Optimist Community Health Trust)

> 'My dental service manager is very corporate, very much a team player. He's finding it extremely hard, because this decision's been made about his service [to make dentists redundant] and he's had to carry out a lot of stuff himself which has been tough. He's coped really well.'
>
> (nurse executive, Pragmatic Community Health Services)

In the second quotation, the dental manager is described in terms that evoke an image of the good bureaucrat, who resists personal interests in his support for organisational goals (Davies 1995).

The good worker was also likely to be sympathetic to the introduction of performance-related pay:

> 'We believe there's a movement of a number of staff to start saying, not necessarily that they want performance related pay, but they want some recognition for the good performers as against the poor performers and so we're going – we don't want them to be demotivated because they think the poor performers get the same and I think that staff are ready for something new; they're getting a bit fed up waiting.'
>
> (chief executive, Pragmatic Community Health Services)

He or she also accepts financial and marketing frameworks, described as 'reality' for their activities:

> 'I think they're coming, many of them are coming to grips with the reality of purchasing and providing and what that really means and how much money is available . . . and we've got some keen practitioners who I think are really trying to get to grips with "what is it I am trying to provide and who are my clients and what should this service look like?"'
>
> (nurse executive, Pragmatic Community Health Services)

And in one vision, the good worker, was too good for the menial tasks mentioned earlier in this chapter:

> ' . . . the Project 2000 folks . . . highly qualified . . . , free, challenging, articulate people who are not being trained to be a bed pan emptier which is great. You can get an NVQ to do that.'
>
> (nurse executive, Optimist Community Health Trust)

Another group of good workers were keen to use computers to facilitate their approach to leg ulcers, and to use them to 'follow trend analysis' of this common problem treated by district nurses (nurse executive, Pragmatic Community Health Services). Despite being, to a certain extent, a new creature, the good worker also preserved some more traditional characteristics; 'good nurses . . . always want to do more' (chief executive, Sceptical Health Services Trust).

> 'I think all of them still have a very strong sense about the personal care delivery and I think that is fundamental to any clinician. . . . I don't think we ever want to lose that because that's actually vital to the patient–clinician relationship.'
>
> (nurse executive, Pragmatic Community Health Services)

The sceptics

The sceptics spoke of such a worker in terms that were not dissimilar. For one, the good worker was 'very keen to change practice' i.e. be open to innovation rather than work traditionally (local manager, Pragmatic Community Health Services). For another the good nurse of the future needed to develop some new survival skills which include the pragmatic adoption of a new discourse. The demonstration or translation of her worth will need to be uttered, in a tongue that, with an appropriate metaphor, has 'general currency' among management. The common, or general currency, of general management appears to be a financial one. This financial talk will be where her plausibility will be located:

> ' . . . she will need to be able [to] articulate in a way which is the general currency amongst management so that her voice is listened to and given credibility.'
>
> (nurse adviser, Pragmatic Community Health Services)

According to a manager who generally identified herself with traditional welfare values, the good health visitor was challenging, partly out of the necessity of scarce resources, the so-called culture of dependency that some users of their service might exhibit:

> 'They expect clients to take on a few things for themselves, which I think is a good thing. The sort of nanny state. I think we have got to encourage people to find out things for themselves and help them to do it.'
>
> (local manager, Pragmatic Community Health Services)

The traditional nurse

Characteristics of the traditional nurse abounded within the interviews along with explanations for their existence. She is everything the general manager is not: she is isolationist, tribal rather than corporate, traditional and unreflective rather than innovative and objectives orientated, hierarchically minded rather than risk-taking. The reasons for some of these were described as deeply rooted in nursing's professional and political culture. For example, one reason for a reluctance among nurses to think corporately was said to stem from the RCN's approach to the introduction of general management in the 1980s. Sections of the nursing workforce were described in terms that appeal to gender and age-related stereotypes:

> 'District Nurses are probably District Nurses for life; they don't leave, they don't move on. The majority of them are – I was going to say mature ladies, but I think that would be really rude – not sort of like 22, 23, 26, they're older than that. They've had a family, they're fairly settled and quite old, so that makes life a little bit more difficult as well.'
>
> (nurse executive, Optimist Community Health Trust)

> 'I suppose they're people in their 30s and 40s.'
>
> (nurse executive, Sceptical Health Services Trust)

This picture was linked to a certain lack of professional development:

> 'I mean for example I went to present some certificates to an ENB [English National Board for Nursing, Midwifery and Health Visiting] elderly course and there were some people there who would never had been on a course for 20 years since their training.'
>
> (nurse executive, Sceptical Health Services Trust)

However, there was said to be another more deep-seated fear among nurses that was to do with ignorance of a professional group that mirrored their own elitist culture:

> ' . . . people who've been trained in clinical care, find it actually quite difficult to cope with management concepts . . . they feel threatened by the management culture because they think it's going to, you know, erode their basic beliefs.'
>
> (chief executive, Optimist Community Health Trust)

Traditional nurses were unreflective; they 'feel they've got to be busy all the time which is a tradition they were brought up in' (nurse executive, Sceptical Health Services Trust). Even when they make complex decisions, they make them almost without realising it:

' . . . what they originally thought was going to happen was that they would be straightforward clinicians and they wouldn't have to make difficult decisions about funds and who received what, and yet all the research shows that they are the people who have been rationing for years and years.'

(nurse executive, Pragmatic Community Health Services)

The final characteristic of the traditional nurse concerns an adherence to hierarchies and rule following:

'Nursing is one of the most autocratically hierarchical professions I've ever come across. Nurses just stop short of standing to attention when the senior nurse walks on the ward.'

(chief executive, Sceptical Health Services Trust)

A certain lack of innovation could be linked to a mentality instilled during nurse training in which it is necessary to 'fairly rigidly follow certain rules, things around drug treatments'. The rigidity that this could give rise to was described by one chief executive as an illness, 'the neurosis about them making a mistake' (chief executive, Pragmatic Community Health Services).

The sceptics

One sceptic attempted to turn the tables to some extent and legitimise the place of the traditional nurse. However, her faltering speech suggests that such a vocabulary was all but unavailable in an organisational and health service culture where other discourses had been developed:

' . . . [much] is forgotten of the general day to day work that is being done, and the sterling work that is being done by not necessarily high-flyers, not necessarily creative people who are giving good standard work; probably above standard, but you know by standard I mean necessary, usual care which is always going to be necessary . . . I find it quite difficult, and this is just personally, just where a good sound solid level will fit in in the future to be honest. You know, someone who is sort of average, bright academically, when I say "average" I mean average and not because the fact that, well, I mean, I mean – no what do I mean?'

(nurse advisor, Pragmatic Community Health Services)

Dead wood

Part of the cultural change within the NHS was said to be a less indulgent attitude towards workers who are underachieving. This was part of a new emphasis on performance, including the championing of performance-related pay. Many managers described the pre-reform service as a comfortable organisation for the complacent, jaded and unmotivated:

'People don't tolerate people who just are not quite as able anymore, not in the same way. I think you'd find 25 percent of the organisation were just – weren't working up to par and were doing all sorts of bizarre things. Nobody ever dealt with them and it was actually quite bizarre and I think people didn't want to deal with it. You know, the NHS was seen as this very happy family.'

(nurse executive, Pragmatic Community Health Services)

One chief executive claimed that nurses were demotivated by the fact that underachieving colleagues received the same pay as themselves and would welcome performance-related pay in some form:

' . . . the so and so you work with who's actually just kind of, you know, just about doing an average job, they're not pulling their weight really or even the ones who aren't even pulling their weight properly at all, still get the annual increments. . . . '

(chief executive, Pragmatic Community Health Services)

For another manager, 'dead wood' included those who, while not necessarily poor performers, had failed to take on the new NHS ethos. Organisational efficiency appeared uppermost in this blend of bodily and botanical metaphors that could be drawn from any number of contemporary organisational essays:

'I would argue that it's the people that are less secure in their positions who perhaps have not taken on board all the changes in the health service and are perhaps not providing the sort of health care that is needed in the current climate that are the most vulnerable and if that means weeding out dead wood, then yes, I would agree that's what's happened because organisations have got to be fitter and leaner.'

(local manager, Sceptical Health Services Trust)

Stress

Managers readily acknowledged that their workforce was under considerable stress due to the accelerating pace of change within the NHS, lower job security, increasing unemployment and social problems among their clients, as well as a range of other factors. Many managers' response to this question often involved listing a range of structural measures introduced to combat stress, such as 'opportunities for counselling' and health and safety policies. A common move was to devalue a *sense* of stress and heavy workload with the argument that no measurable change was apparent. In one passage, which I would like to deal with at length, a chief executive accounted for the stress of her staff through a series of rhetorical moves:

'I find this quite an interesting one because people do feel stressed and people feel they are working harder, but in lots of ways when we've made changes, we've cut things out as well and so it's very hard for me to say whether technically people are working harder than they were before.'

(chief executive, Pragmatic Community Health Services)

By introducing her response as 'interesting', immediately a certain detachment is created and stress becomes an object of knowledge. Then, by contrasting what people 'feel' with the concept of measurability, and casting doubt on the 'technical' reality of a cause of that stress, it begins to be marginalised.

'I think what happens in health care is the kind of people you get in are the kind of people who want to do a good job and whatever level of resource you gave them, there'd be people like me; I feel stressed because I work very hard, but I know that I make that stress for myself by taking on extra things and always wanting to do better.'

(ibid.)

This further move is to suggest that in some respects people are responsible for creating their own stress. To include herself among such individuals and to link stress to aspiration adds authority to what might otherwise appear as overt victim-blaming. Then there is the assertion that stress is intrinsic to the job: 'sometimes we can't take the stress out of our jobs, partly because the jobs are stressful . . . that's a feature of the job'. In addition the suggestion that stress levels are volatile acts rhetorically to attenuate it:

'I don't know how the staff at the front-line feel as a whole, because although I ask a lot my feeling is that it changes almost from week to week.'

(ibid.)

The argument that it is a result of a local and incomplete orientation rather than a global, organisational view functions in a similar way:

' . . . if you put forward 20 developments you get six, but the people who didn't get the 14 feel fed up.'

(ibid.)

Stress can also result from 'one or two people [who] just have really unreasonable expectations' who, like bad apples, 'then have an effect on the rest of the team'.

At the end of this rhetorically accomplished passage, the addressee almost cannot help viewing staff stress as less distressing.

AUTONOMY AND TRADITION

A central characteristic of the construction of the modern self is its autonomy. Kant argued that the Enlightenment was a process that had the potential to release humanity from 'a certain state that makes us accept someone else's authority' when the use of our own reason is called for (Rabinow 1984: 34). Through philosophers, including Descartes and Hume, the figure of the autonomous human subject emerged who would 'take nothing and no authority for granted whose content and strictures had not been subjected to rigorous examination, and that had not withstood the test of "clarity and distinctness"' (Benhabib 1990: 109). A version of the self was constructed over a relatively short historical period that was stripped of cultural, ethical and religious dimensions, and remained as 'a pure subject of knowledge' or consciousness or mind. Correspondingly, the object of knowledge was reduced to 'matters of fact' or 'sensations' and 'concepts'. In a sense this modern self found itself disembodied and disconnected from the world and so was faced with the task of reconnecting the representations within its consciousness to those without. Two solutions tended to be adopted: either a privileging of the direct and immediate evidence of the senses, an approach which came to be known as empiricism, or a belief that the rationality of the creator or the harmony between mind and nature would ensure a correspondence between the two orders of representations (rationalism). Hence for the last two hundred years, the task faced by those concerned with the generation of knowledge has involved addressing the question of adequate representation. The mind has been seen as 'the mirror of nature' (Rorty 1980). This picture of knowledge involves unproblematic understandings of the self, the object of knowledge, the relationship between the two and the language with which we might designate and describe these objects.

These three notions have been subject to strong critique. First, the notion of the transparent knowing subject has been refuted by those like Marx and Engels (1969) and Hegel (1977) who have argued that the spectator view of the self does not take into account the subterranean contextual influences of history and culture upon ideas which are thought to be clear and distinct. Similarly, Freud has shown that the self is not transparent to itself but is controlled by desires, needs and forces which shape both its ideas and their organisation (Freud 1953). The second critique concerns the relationship between the modern subject and the object of knowledge which some have characterised as one of domination (Heidegger 1962; Nietzsche 1994). Modern knowledge divides the world into the realms of appearance and essence and the spectator self into a similar dualism of body and mind. This leads to a conception of being as presence, in other words, what is available to, or present to, the consciousness of the subject. This conception reduces the heterogeneity of appearances into whatever is present to the subject and in turn makes available the possibility of their control by that subject. A homogeneity is imposed, in this way, upon objects of knowledge by the very unit of Western thought, the 'concept' (Benhabib 1990: 111).

It is possible to understand the managers in this research as in a similar predicament to that ascribed to the modern self. First, because of the managerial claim to a morality based on effectiveness and efficiency they are open to the charge that subconscious, historical and political drives and influences have been erased from their self-descriptions. Second, because of their conception of and search for largely value-free objective knowledge as a basis for understanding the workings of their organisation and workforce and for acting, they can be seen as disconnected from the embodied and heterogeneous knowledge and experience of health care and as imposing a certain dominating organisation upon it. Third, because of a view of language as the transparent equivalent of 'clear and distinct' thought, the power of domination and manipulation already present in categorical thinking is undeclared. Their discourse relies on the possibility of innocent representation and autonomy of thought and action.

Autonomy, in the discourse of the managers, appeared as the mirror image of the 'traditional' mentality that they often attributed to nurses. As we have seen, managers characterised the traditional mode of thought as involving a reliance upon authority and unthinking adherence to long-established rules and routines. Managers in this study prized autonomy for themselves and their organisations but, paradoxically, they spoke of a need to curb the activities of doctors who were also exhibiting this attribute. In introducing and promoting the NHS reforms, the UK government emphasised the freedom and self-determination apparently on offer to management teams who were willing to join the scheme. These freedoms included the ability to set their own terms and conditions of employment and to configure their services in ways that they considered appropriate to their local situations as well as being the type of services that they might want to develop. No longer would decisions have to be ratified by successively distant committees of bureaucrats in health authorities and at regional level. This freedom, which included an ability to raise loans, within certain restrictions, was likely to be particularly attractive to the managers of the new community units whose budgets traditionally had been in danger from overspending hospital units. In place of complex bureaucratic relationships, small boards of directors were offered apparently unprecedented opportunity to run their own affairs.

Senior managers described their willingness to accept the responsibility that they associated with autonomy in a metaphorical language that enacted a certain conventional drama of effectiveness, a drama which MacIntyre considers 'a masquerade of social control', 'a theatre of illusions' (MacIntyre 1985: 75, 77):

> ' . . . the buck stops here with me and my Board. There's no hiding place.'
> (chief executive, Optimist Community Health Trust)

For MacIntyre, assertions of effectiveness purport to give information about reality but do no more than express the attitudes and beliefs of those who utter them. 'Managerial effectiveness' functions in a similar way to how talk about

God has been understood, '[i]t is the name of a fictitious, but believed-in reality, appeal to which disguises certain other realities' (MacIntyre 1985: 76). MacIntyre claims that among these other realities is the desire to persuade and manipulate.

Managers themselves often drew a distinction between the freedoms that the NHS reforms allowed, which they eventually realised were limited, and the energetic and imaginative mentality that they engendered. However, this did not cause them to doubt their own effectiveness. In a sense this supported and augmented their belief in their ability to bring about change. Again, the figurative language appeals to an Enlightenment aspiration for humanity to be 'master of its destiny':

> 'The change too was of course that to an extent [as] masters of your own destiny you could make changes happen but the big shift was the belief that you could change it.'
>> (nurse executive, Optimist Community Health Trust)

In Chapter 1, we saw that management writers Peters and Waterman emphasised that a *sense* of self-determination could have considerable influence on an employee's motivation (Peters and Waterman 1982). They argued that the effective manager is aware of this and uses this knowledge as part of his or her strategy for managing. In this study managers often referred to concerted efforts to foster this same belief among the nursing workforce. There is a certain contradiction in the language with which managers spoke of these efforts with its mixture of constraint, 'pushing' and freedom:

> ' . . . we pushed that feeling of "we're a Trust, we're independent" through to our staff.'
>> (nurse executive, Optimist Community Health Trust)

> ' . . . we have started pushing financial control towards the staff to give them more control over things.'
>> (chief executive, Pragmatic Community Health Services)

> 'The important thing is to make the GPs believe that they have some control over the processes and if they believe that then they are not going to pull away.'
>> (nurse executive, Pragmatic Community Health Services)

The contradiction is appropriate because, certainly in the first two of the above examples, managers set the overall context within which they granted a limited degree of choice to their employees. This is perhaps the best way of understanding the talk of, particularly nurse executives, who spoke of a desire to encourage nurses to be 'far more autonomous in the way that they practise' (nurse executive, Pragmatic Community Health Services). This appeal to coveted notions of professionalism within nursing, ignores the confined nature of the autonomy that is possible in this situation. In fact, it could be argued that the 'pushing of financial control' towards staff who are directly involved in care delivery represents a cynical delegation of the working out of the details of highly sensitive financial cutbacks. The overall effect could be quite the opposite of empowering. The third example refers to a discussion about the possibility that local GP fundholders may, if legislation should permit them, directly employ the community nurses presently employed by Community Trusts and thus possibly jeopardise the financial viability of organisations like the ones involved in this study. The manager who is speaking is suggesting that the relationship between Trust managers and GPs needs to be carefully managed so that, should the legislation change, GPs would not wish to assert their independence. Granting them some control now may avert the later situation in which the Trust would lose all control.

The 'socially beneficial autonomy' (Pollitt 1993: 10) claimed by managers for their own decisions and activities can be seen as a late imitation of the clinical judgement and freedom established by professionals such as doctors. That the managerial claim is a derivation from other claims to authority can be problematic because individual clinicians' access to this source of autonomy is now no longer legitimate. They are to subjugate autonomous activity to the overall authority of the organisation's managers.

'What you need is greater powers for the FHSA [Family Health Service Authority] to deal with the recalcitrant GPs and there is the odd GP around who is, quite frankly, clueless about a lot of the stuff we do and even if we spent hours and hours talking to them they wouldn't understand it and they would need some control.'

(chief executive, Pragmatic Community Health Services)

'A couple of surgeons are still trying to do their own thing. So we've imposed, and I do mean imposed, quota systems for operating.'

(chief executive, Sceptical Health Services Trust)

In these quotations, the clinicians who are exercising what in other contexts would be termed autonomy are described negatively by these managers as being irresponsible, 'clueless', 'recalcitrant' or 'trying to do their own thing'.

The notion of the autonomy of the individual has been examined by postmodern thinkers (see Chapter 2). In addition, professional medical autonomy has been called into question by, among others, Celia Davies who argues that each clinician–patient encounter, which is the image of the exercise of professional autonomy, is sustained and made possible only by largely invisible work carried out by, for example, nurses and clerical staff (Davies 1995). Talk of autonomy, then, whether by managers or clinicians, can be seen as the expressive activity suggested by MacIntyre, and even perhaps as carrying what Nietzsche has termed the 'will to power' (Nietzsche 1967).

In the texts of nurses, we can see an expression of the tension between the discourse of professional autonomy and the experience of control by management and the strategies that are used to reconcile the two. These texts are discussed in the next chapter.

8 Morality and self-sacrifice: the nurses' comments

In the design of the RCN study, the gathering of nurses' written comments was supplementary to the main objective of numerically measuring their job satisfaction. Numerically speaking, nurses were provided with a residue of 3.5 inches of blank paper within which to respond to the invitation to comment. Nurses responded by creating a particular kind of space shaped by powerful enactment of their subjectivities, often set in contrast to descriptions of rising forces that they saw within their organisations or in society as a whole. The strongly worded quotations of this chapter are not atypical of these comments. Anger, frustration, outrage and bitterness were common. Comments that supported managerial perspectives and organisational change appeared, but were rare in the extreme. The comments as a whole are striking partly because they contrast with both the discourse of managers involved in the study and with many of the 'official' discourses of nursing leaders discussed in Chapter 4.

Interestingly, comments made by practice nurses who are employed by General Practitioners showed certain differences and similarities to their colleagues employed within Trusts. They were certainly more upbeat in terms of their assessment of their working conditions, many making comparisons to previous work as health authority employees, but, as we shall see, their view of contemporary changes in health care and declarations of their own guiding ethos are little different to those of other nurses.

WHO, WHEN AND WHERE? A BACKGROUND TO THE QUESTIONNAIRE COMMENTS

Table 8.1 shows the number of nurses that wrote comments during the three years of the study and in the various organisations. For the purposes of the analysis offered in this chapter, with one exception, little distinction is drawn between sites and years. Comments varied in length between a sentence and up to two sides of closely written text, attached to the original questionnaire. Practice nurses from the four study areas are included with their local Trust. The job titles of nurses who commented are shown in Table 8.2. The three years of the study are combined. Middle managers employed in the Trusts were included

Table 8.1 Nurses commenting: all years and all Trusts

Year	Optimist Community Health Trust and Brick-built Hospital Trust	Absolute Trust	Sceptical Health Services Trust	Pragmatic Community Health Services	All Trusts
1	141	86	54	88	369
2	130	withdrew	57	92	279
3	115		44	79	238
All years	386	86	155	259	886

Table 8.2 Job title and number of nurses commenting

Job title	Number
Practice nurse	198
District nurse	140
Health visitor	177
Nursing auxiliary	82
All trained hospital staff*	83
Enrolled nurse	60
Community staff nurse	41
Schools nurse	25
Middle manager	24
Other	56
All nurses	886

* One of the Trusts operated four small community hospitals

in the study of job satisfaction as well as in the interview study of managers so that their morale could be compared to other staff. I have not included their comments in this chapter's analysis.

A CARING/CASH DUALISM

In Chapter 2, we saw how one of the characteristic approaches of deconstruction involved the examination of a text's dualisms. This can make explicit a hierarchical privilege given to one side of such dualisms and enable a questioning of the whole basis of the hierarchy. Following this tendency, I would now like to examine how nurses wrote about themselves, their activities and their priorities, very often in relation to those they described as typifying management. It is through this dualistic device, I will argue, that they aligned their subjectivity with the moral supremacy of caring.

Critical attitudes towards managers and administrators have a long history among nurses (Mercer 1979). A great many nurses involved in this study described many aspects of what they tended to set up as a dichotomy between management and themselves in terms of values and priorities. They often did this by means of a range of 'us–them' dualisms. The majority of these dualisms opposed 'care' to 'money', but other dualisms created different dimensions of an alienation many nurses described. 'Caring' was accorded not only a moral but an epistemological privilege. In other words, not only was this discursive structure the means by which nurses adopted a position of moral superiority, but they tended to describe the knowledge that it gave access to as of a more real and authoritative nature than the more abstract knowledge which they associated with managers' reports and 'statistics'. This closely woven series of dualisms enacts how one aspect of nurses' subjectivity was constituted by combining discourses of moral value and of empiricism, an assertion of the privilege of the direct evidence of the senses.

I have tried to resist the temptation to write about nurses and managers in the same dualistic ways that they appeared to speak about each other because this would be to collude, in a sense, with the mirage of stability and homogeneity attempted by both discourses. I will suggest later that both nurses and managers jump out of any stable subjectivity that either I or they might invent for themselves. As others have argued, subjectivity can be understood not as a given or as a deep characteristic of the self but as something that needs constantly to be performed and maintained (Garfinkel 1967). However, it is hard not to comment that in some respects nurses' discourse gave rise to a subjectivity which was strikingly different to that adopted by managers. Managers tended to assert the epistemology of the overview, with its detachment, that lent them an ability to penetrate to the reality of the situation and make, effectively, better decisions. However, managers also questioned the moral capability of some of their clinical staff to abandon traditional mentalities and face up to 'realistic' financial constraints and responsibilities. Some nurses explicitly identified their work and values as 'traditional' while managers spoke of themselves as bringers of modernity and radical change, as I described in Chapter 7. The power of successful rhetoric is such that both groups can present these clashing discourses in a way that we as readers are persuaded by both. Many nurses identified the threat to 'caring values' as a new phenomenon, and this too was reflected in the words of managers who, as I have tried to show, took the NHS reforms as a central reference point in their world view.

The reader of the nurses' comments would initially be struck by their tone of moral outrage. A similar atmosphere of outrage often featured in the staff meetings that I attended in the Trusts. Perhaps it is consistent with the subjectivities performed by managers and nurses that the former should adopt the language of solidarity with their organisation, of control, of the rationality of the statement based on scepticism or observation and that the latter, lacking this organisational identification and not using this vocabulary, had learnt to draw upon a moral discourse to characterise their subjectivity.

Although such comments were made by nurses in all four study areas, relatively twice as many comments were made by nurses from Optimist Community Health

Trust, and particularly from community hospital staff in that Trust, in the first year of the research. These comments of strong disaffection were rarities in the second year of the survey in that area. This was the only instance of a major change over time. The reason for this is unclear. When I asked nurses at a staff meeting in the area if they had any explanation, some suggested that the need to 'let off steam' had passed while others said they had been too dispirited to offer a similar comment a second time.

The following statement achieves much of its effect through the use of dualism. In it, a nurse expresses the much voiced belief that financial priorities have taken over from the concerns of patient care (a theme that is discussed later):

> 'Patient comfort is obviously not the main concern of the hierarchy, as long as they can keep within budget, that's all that seems to matter. . . . '
> (staff nurse, Optimist Community Health Trust)

In this statement 'Patient comfort' and keeping 'within budget' are set up as opposites in which the former term is implicitly, but clearly, privileged as the more legitimate, authentic concern and activity. 'Keep[ing] within budget' is described as a supplementary concern that has usurped its proper position. This kind of criticism of usurpation or reversal of values is frequently made in nurses' comments. Keeping within budget is, through the use of this dualism, described as having no bearing at all on patient comfort and can be rhetorically dismissed.

The use of the term 'the hierarchy' with its suggestion of power, distance, bureaucracy and impersonality, also contrasts with the highly personal and immediate 'Patient comfort'. Not only are these managers nameless, they are titleless too. This characterisation of management, along with the emphasis of 'obviously' and 'that's all that seems to matter', make the outrage and hostility of this comment unmistakeable. In fact, the dynamic of hyperbole commandeers the utterance; in the first line the patient is of secondary concern to management while a line later, the patient does not figure at all. This comment, which is characteristic of a great many nurses' comments is clearly very different to the utterances of the managers who rarely, though sometimes, made such frank use of emotionally charged rhetoric. The comment continues:

> 'Money is also being wasted on such things as plastic drink mats, promoting the Community Trust! which have no benefit to the patients whatsoever.'
> (staff nurse, Optimist Community Health Trust)

If the hierarchy's obvious lack of concern for patient comfort identifies it as alien, its choice of what to actually spend on is even more out of tune with the patient-centred priority that nurses often identified with. Other nurses similarly contrasted expenditure on computer equipment with money that could have been spent on direct patient care. This statement of equivalences and alternatives shows us that nurses could, as we shall soon see, attack and simultaneously use utilitarian notions.

A further aspect of the nurses' view of management priorities is expressed as a dualism between the theoretical or administrative and the practical:

> 'I feel that management are far too concerned with statistics and complicated paperwork, and as long as these are in order, they really aren't concerned about the patient's well-being.'
>
> (staff nurse, Optimist Community Health Trust)

The main point in this statement appears to be not so much that statistics and paperwork might be unreliable indicators of patient well-being, but that they stand for a specific frame of reference, one that is characterised by a distance from care delivery and that is 'complicated' as opposed to one that is direct and practical. In extraordinary similarity to the previous comment, the writer suggests that the indicators themselves have usurped the place in managers' concerns that should rightfully be occupied by *the thing itself* to which the indicators testify. The dualism tears apart any connection between the 'paperwork' and the patient so that whether the paperwork is 'in order' (an abstract bureaucratic term) or not can be described as having no connection to the well-being of real patients.

Another hospital based nurse expands on the same point, adding the suggestion that such a complicated outlook is a new intrusion into nursing:

> 'I'm dissatisfied with the "simple is best" attitude in nursing being replaced by "Let's complicate, high tech." attitude coming in. Empathy, bedside manner, care. These words are being replaced by customer, computer, audit, budget.'
>
> (staff nurse, Optimist Community Health Trust)

I have already examined this comment in Chapter 3 as an example of my approach to textual analysis. Suffice it to say here that its main structure centres around two dualisms. Both are enacted by contrasting two different types of language. This suggests that this nurse is aware of changes in language use within her organisation and how these may be linked to overall values or organisational culture, what she terms 'attitude'. It is because of this link that she can contrast the traditional, 'empathy, bedside manner, care', along with their associations of intimacy and humanity, with the words 'customer, computer, audit, budget' which have wholly different connotations. As in the previous quotation, complication is characterised as something negative which can be both contrasted with the principle of 'simple is best' and associated with the 'high-tech' computer. The physical and emotional world of practical action is contrasted with a numerically dominated, abstract realm.

In all the above quotations, and in many others, the commenters manage our reading of financial concern by constantly rhetorically contrasting it with the moral worthiness of patient care. Any positive connection between the two is erased by this device.

Some nurses also opposed their orientation to forces operating within their own profession. In comments that called upon a discourse of the impersonality of modernity, the space occupied by bureaucratic managers was expanded to implicate the whole of society including nursing's own leaders:

> 'Modern society seems to be drowning in technology and bureaucracy. Patient care has been put in the hands of highly qualified managers, most of whom have had no contact with actual patients/clients.'
>
> (staff nurse, Optimist Community Health Trust)

> 'I am increasingly getting the feeling that 100% isn't enough and that courses, CATS points, nursing diploma's etc. etc. are more important than our patients. While I appreciate that we all need training can't there be a balance – what are we there for, to care for our patients or to wander around waving our pieces of paper for courses and talking in the latest jargon. This is what I now feel the UKCC [United Kingdom Central Council for Nursing, Midwifery and Health Visiting] thinks is important.'
>
> (practice nurse, Sceptical Health Services Trust)

In the second comment, expanding educational opportunities (or pressures) are contrasted with the effort put into caring, '100% isn't enough'. The highly rhetorical figure of the nurse 'wander[ing] around waving . . . pieces of paper for courses and talking in the latest jargon' effects a separation of the notion of nurse education from 'caring for our patients' which is the *telos* of nursing. The nurse is 'wandering around' rather than delivering care and carrying the paper that is consistently used by commenting nurses to symbolise the antithetical realm of the nonphysical and administrative. Through these rhetorical devices, the writer can present what might be considered an extreme view as 'a balance'.

Table 8.3 summarises an approach to the types of dualism that can be derived from the comments. The following five categories were devised after examination of passages in which nurses described their own concerns or values alongside a contrasting set of concerns which they attributed to management. Only in a very few comments did nurses discriminate between different levels of management. In these cases senior management were singled out for particular comment. The first element of the dualism summarises how they wrote about their own characteristic concerns; the second is what they associated with management.

Table 8.4 goes on to give examples, drawn from the first year's comments, of the categories outlined in Table 8.3. Each line identifies the two opposing values that are contrasted in a single comment. In some cases one comment falls into two of the Table 8.3 categories. From Table 8.4 it can be seen that nurses strongly identified themselves with a concern for patient 'comfort' and 'welfare'

Table 8.3 Categories of dualism in nurses' comments

1	patient care – finance;
2	manual work – nonmanual work;
3	work for patients – work for the trust;
4	human concern for employees – accounting concern for finance;
5	practical – theoretical.

Table 8.4 Analysis of comments on management

Nurses' concerns	Managers' concerns	Category
care	'profit and loss'	1
patient comfort	being 'within budget'	1
patient care	'money is god and clerical work second'	1,2
employees as people and welfare of clients	a 'business', saving money	1,4
patients and staff	saving money and 'getting a good name for themselves'	1,3
patient care	'posh offices'	1,3
patients' well-being	'statistics and complicated paperwork'	5
contact with clients	'highly qualified'	5
communication	'waffle'	5
matron was 'approachable, respected, there for her staff and knew what was going on'	'too aloof'	5
identifying client needs	promoting the Trust	3
'in touch with reality'	'cuckoo land'	5
'simple is best'	'let's complicate, high-tech.'	5
'empathy, bedside manner, care'	'customer, computer, audit, budget'	1,5
'common-sense hands'	'thoughtful eyes'	5
expenditure on:		
nursing staff	computer equipment	2,5
damaged floor	plastic coasters	3
basic equipment ('for patient comfort')	'outward shows'	3

and the comments, discussed on pages 142 and 143, suggest that they felt strongly that it was the proper priority of their organisation.

So far, this analysis has conveyed little of the dynamic way that nurses might constantly renegotiate their subjectivity within a situation in which they struggle to maintain power. Questions of how individuals take up, negotiate, or resist discourse and how resistance might be generated and sustained will be addressed in the following section as well as in Chapter 9.

Exceptional exceptions

Although very few nurses from any of the Trust areas made positive comments about management, those that were ventured (by three nurses during the course of the whole study) provide the opportunity to ask, if not to answer the question, what prompted them? Were these nurses' managers different in some way to those described by other nurses or is it the nurses who made positive comments who are different and, furthermore, can a study of these few exceptional positive comments shed any light on the general rule of negativity? Positive views tended to be strongly worded, standing out sharply from a background of adverse comment. I include two of these comments. The first comes from a staff nurse in Optimist Community Health Trust, a Trust where nurses' comments were characterised by harshly critical comments about management.

> 'The amount of support I receive from my managers is enormous. I have been given a lot of opportunities to attend courses with study time and financial backing. . . . Career advice has been offered and I have been encouraged to reach for promotion. Management style within the hospital is dynamic with clear aims. Understandable rationales are given for tasks requested. There is also an air of "openness" and new ideas are also welcomed and encouraged. There is plenty of room for personal development. I certainly feel a sense of loyalty to the hospital, colleagues, patients and management.'
>
> (staff nurse, Optimist Community Health Trust)

The second comment is from Pragmatic Community Health Services:

> 'The unit general manager is approachable, dynamic and motivating: she knows many of the staff and appreciates us for the work we do. There is a good communication system for transfer of news between management and field staff.'
>
> (district nurse, Pragmatic Community Health Services)

The strength of the difference between these comments and virtually every other comment did prompt discussion in the research unit about whether the questionnaires containing them might be 'plants' by managers with a mischievous sense of humour!

SPLIT SUBJECTIVITY: CARING AND EXPLOITATION IN THE TEXTS

The ways in which 'official' nursing discourses have at times placed caring at the centre of talk about nursing have been described in Chapter 4. Nurses in this study appeared to do the same although the way that they achieved this was less theoretically orientated and framed almost exclusively in problematic terms.

The study of discourse provides the notion of split subjectivity, which can usefully open up the texts of the nurses, for many appeared to be negotiating between a discourse of caring as morally worthwhile, intrinsically satisfying and even empowering, and an alternative discourse of exploitation and dis-empowerment in the workplace. A discursive strategy that might reconcile these two positions lay in adopting the position of personal sacrifice. Because nurses could link their activity with a moral orientation, their talk of individual judgement could avoid the charge of professional elitism. This was possible partly because, since what MacIntyre describes as the failure of the Enlighten-ment project to justify morality in terms of appeals to a universal reason, morality has been understood as belonging to the realm of personal judgements (MacIntyre 1985). Within this moral position of self-sacrifice, the exercise of individual judgement about standards of care can be understood as a point of resistance to the power of management to measure and control their activity.

In order to explore this we can first look at how nurses constructed 'caring' in their texts. This account is drawn from the one hundred comments made about this topic. Second, we can consider ways in which constraints upon caring were figured and resisted.

Often nurses adopted the discourses of vocation and duty that, as we have seen in Chapter 4, many of the profession's leaders have been reluctant to accept in favour of more professionalised discourses. Nurses described caring in strongly personal terms. They described themselves as bringing to the encounter with the patient a personal commitment to helping and supporting and a belief that particular individuals had a need for as well as an entitlement to the service that they offered.

Within the act of caring, nurses appeared acutely aware that care could vary in quality and that good quality caring demanded, above all, adequate time. Adequate resources, training and qualified nurses were also described as necessary by some. Determining what high quality care looked like was a matter of individ-ual judgement, referred to sometimes as 'professional judgement' and as an outworking of the personal standards of the nurse. It resulted in emotional satisfaction for both patient and nurse. However, descriptions of situations where satisfaction was *not* the outcome tended to dominate talk of care. In these situa-tions the outcome was stress and distress for the nurses involved. Nurses pointed to lack of time as the main obstacle to these high standards of care and went on to make a distinction between their 'own time' and their paid working hours. They frequently cited the encroachment into their personal time of work activity as an example of the personal sacrifice that they offered in an attempt to avoid what they saw as poor quality or incomplete care. Administrative duties were seen as the antithesis to care delivery and were frequently identified as a cause of time constraints. The practicality of care delivery was contrasted with and seen to be under threat not only from management but from the profession's own leaders' and educators' attempts to theorise or complicate it. As we have seen, caring was constructed as an activity of high moral value and contrasted with financial concerns which were seen as less morally valuable and even morally dubious.

Caring as commitment

If caring was to be successfully pictured as a moral activity it would not fit entirely within usual occupational limits. Many nurses characterised their activities by appealing to a discourse of vocation which for some crossed the boundary between the private and public spheres:

> 'I am doing the job I had always wanted to do, caring for people that needed caring or a helping hand. . . . '
>
> (nursing auxiliary)

> 'I came into nursing to look after people and at the end of the day if the patient goes home satisfied with the care he or she has received, then I feel happy.'
>
> (staff nurse)

> 'The care that patients/clients get is due to the commitment of the individual nurses including myself. I like to do my job to the best of my ability and put myself out in order to do it, i.e. come in early, do without lunch etc.'
>
> (health visitor)

> 'Each day I aim to do my job to 100% of my capabilities to ensure my patients' well-being and happiness, and then return home to do the same for the rest of my family.'
>
> (practice nurse)

Surprisingly, the basis of practice was generally described in terms of personal qualities rather than as professional training. Training could be called upon, however, as evidence of the legitimacy of direct care activity:

> 'Since I filled in the previous questionnaire a type of "case-work plan" has been introduced where I work. This has altered greatly my ability to cope with what I was trained for – namely "care of the sick". I spend increasing amounts of time writing – whilst my auxiliaries care and "hands on" my patients. This is the reason I am much less satisfied with my work than I was when last I answered your questionnaire. I resent the fact that new fangled time-wasters come between me and my proper nursing training and etiquette. I like writing but not when my patients need practical help.'
>
> (Marie Curie nurse)

In this comment, 'proper' and the slightly old-fashioned 'etiquette' contrast with 'new fangled'. Such a move allows nursing training and practice to align with tradition and propriety while other, possibly administrative acts, align with the faddish and trivial. The purpose of nurse training being described as 'care of the sick' acts to persuade the reader of its direct and almost timeless quality and status.

Need for and entitlement to nursing

Caring involved an encounter between the personally committed nurse and the patient who also brought a personal attribute, and particular moral status, that of having 'need'. Nurses expressed a strong sense of urgency regarding this need (see emphasis in the first quotation below) yet need also appeared, paradoxically, to be something defined and detected by nurses as in the comments below and particularly in the argument that certain families 'need' 'professional support and guidance':

'As a student I have more opportunity to spend longer time with patients/ families, time that THEY NEED.'

(district nursing student; original emphasis)

'Approx. 1/3 of my caseload comprises of families of concern (various reasons) who need extra HV support and it is a constant struggle to provide them with the professional support/guidance which they need and are entitled to.'

(health visitor)

'Some of the children I care for would benefit from and have the right to be cared for by paediatric trained nurses.'

(school nurse)

Some nurses wrote about their patients' 'right' and 'entitlement' to receive care, as in the second and third comment above. This aligned nurses' identities with two discrete but associated discourses. The first can be described broadly as a welfare discourse, a discourse which reverberates with the founding ethos of the UK National Health Service itself. Within this discourse, entitlement has moral associations but can be considered a specific reference to formal citizenship entitlements springing from the payment of national insurance contributions. The second is a more overtly moral discourse which, particularly when we discuss further passages, can be considered deontological, calling upon notions of the supreme value of each individual (Seedhouse 1993). Deontologists argue that each human life has an intrinsic value which cannot be reduced by illness or disability. Because of this, utilitarian arguments that are based upon setting measurable equivalents between the different benefits of health care, involved, for example in the notion of QALYs (Quality Adjusted Life Years) (Maynard 1993), are rejected. Some deontologists might claim that any value judgements about the rationing of health care are unacceptable and that the only appropriate basis for rationing would be a random one (Seedhouse 1993). An implicit, and often explicit, deontology characterised many of the comments by nurses contrasting with the largely utilitarian discourse of the managers. It may be this fundamental difference in ethical stance that made nurses appear so irrational to managers whose most urgent work involved determining equivalents and comparisons in the use of apparently fixed resources. In fact nurses often contrasted 'patients' needs' with 'saving money', letting the comment that the latter had taken precedence in managerial attention stand as a sign of a declining moral climate within their organisations.

Individual judgement about the standard of care as a point of resistance

Nurses wrote about the care they delivered as revolving around a number of personal decisions and judgements rather than, for example conforming to pre-established criteria. This was possible because they had already, discursively, established both the moral basis of their work and their own legitimacy as moral agents. Decisions made about caring, then, could be described, unproblematically, as originating from the realm of the personal, and, to a lesser extent, from professional judgement. It was this characterisation that so frustrated management in its drive for nurses to work in a rational, formalised way. These judgements could be the one site where nurses had the possibility of exercising power. The criteria for quality and for decisions about care were nearly always described in the language of personal feeling and judgement:

'I hope I give an extremely high standard of care.'

(health visitor)

'. . . not able to give quality of care I think patient needs.'

(district nurse)

'I like to think that I give the patients a good quality of care, but the pressures of the job sometimes make me anxious that perhaps I am rushing things too much and not giving the time to the patients that they need.'

(district nurse)

Yet, surprisingly, the great majority of comments about caring described not a situation of autonomy and satisfaction but one of frustration:

'[I am] always aiming to offer the patients in the care of my team a high standard of quality care. I am now struggling to continue my standard of care.'

(district nurse)

'Nurses desperately trying to maintain a high standard of care to patients but all done with unpaid overtime.'

(district nurse)

The single nurse who wrote about formalised outcomes and linked standards of care to an organisational rather than personal initiative, provided the only notable exception to this tendency:

'Overall trust status has centred thinking and improved standards of care with more emphasis on outcomes of care.'

(health visitor)

The personal sacrifices made in order to care

The personal judgement and personal moral standards that nurses brought to caring appeared rarely to bring satisfaction or to empower them. Nurses frequently emphasised the personal sacrifice in terms of time they worked to achieve a standard of care that they judged necessary. Nurses could be described as caught in a split subjectivity. It would be inconsistent with the type of moral identity they enacted to object or refuse to carry work into hours beyond those which were financially rewarded; nevertheless, nurses also wrote about continued exploitation. As a way of negotiating a position that accounted for both subjectivities, moral agent and employee, many adopted a discourse of self-sacrifice. This could intensify the moral quality of their subjectivity because it gave evidence that their actions were not self-interested and could render the injustice of their exploitation all the more outrageous because their moral sensitivity rendered them particularly vulnerable to abuse. This move also allowed an alignment of their interests with that of their patients, in a claim that their employers had abandoned human values. This subject position, however, was wide enough to accommodate a range of stances, for example the following two comments featured frank anger:

'The community trust is a business, managers are no longer concerned about employees as people while the welfare of clients comes secondary to saving money.'

(health visitor)

'GPs now financially rather than care orientated. . . . Recently GPs insisted on changing our appointment system to 5 minute units which has put a lot of extra pressure on us and receptionists. We are seen now seen as just money makers.'

(practice nurse)

Others took more ambivalent positions which comprised both acceptance and refusal to accept the situation:

'The care that patients/clients get is due to the commitment of the individual nurses including myself. I like to do my job to the best of my ability and put myself out in order to do it i.e. come in early, do without lunch etc.'

(health visitor)

'I never mind working into my own time but if I did I would not be able to give the patient care I feel would be necessary for long term well-being of patient.'

(nursing auxiliary)

'I do a lot of overtime in order to finish my work and give the patients I visit the care they are entitled to have, but of course do not get paid for this.'

(clinical nurse specialist)

'I spend a lot of my own personal time with patients i.e. I always run late in order to give them the care they need – I don't mind – because I do have a lot of job satisfaction however – I should not HAVE to regularly use my own time to give proper care.'

(nursing auxiliary; original emphasis)

The moral and the dubious

As we have seen in the section on dualism (pp. 140–146), many nurses asserted a strong contrast between the moral value of caring for people and the lesser, and even dubious, consideration for financial matters which they identified with the realm of management. These kinds of comment made in the first year of the study, in the months immediately following the introduction of the reforms, were more frequent and vehement in their language than those of subsequent years and were, as previously mentioned, particularly concentrated among those nurses employed in Optimist Community Health Trust.

This dualism allowed them, by firmly associating their subjectivity with caring, and by recording the personal sacrifices involved in delivering care, to enhance their moral position:

'Numbers, finances and balancing books is becoming more important than people. The organisation doesn't really CARE for its workforce and yet the worker can have given a lifetime of commitment to the NHS. . . . '

(health visitor; original emphasis)

'The world of business has definitely taken over, and as well as not giving as much time to the patients as we would like, there is a lack of caring for us as the carers. . . . '

(district nurse)

While a small number of nurses included acknowledgement of 'financial viability', most who wrote about this maintained a strong hierarchy between 'patients' and 'pounds'. One nurse expressed an uncompromising view that underlies many of the comments made in the first year. She suggests that the need of the human individual completely transcends any financial orientation:

> 'The amount of services and equipment provided to the patients have to be considered first so that we won't be over the budget, I think is petty. I think we should look at the care services available first rather than discussing how much money it will incur. Working within budget policy is unapplicable and inappropriate in caring for elderly/mentally handicapped and or physically handicapped clients.'
>
> (staff nurse)

At the staff meetings nurses often appeared to adopt a posture of fatalism:

> An HV (Health visitor) said, 'No one has personally said [this] but an ethos is dripping down and the ethos is money. Its always money.' 'Is there anything that you can do, faced with all this?' I asked. 'We're pretty much pawns in some of this. You can't fight against the power of money.'
>
> (field notes, November 1992, Pragmatic Community Health Services)

Finally, the atmosphere of increasing financial constraint along with an increasing prominence given to the vocabulary of finance suggested, for some, a fantasy of an NHS that had abandoned even the rhetoric of health care and, one might suspect from the exaggeration of the comment below, was in the process of turning itself into a corporate bank:

> 'Money is the first and last consideration – no mention of patient care in any new NHS proposals. It is "how much will it cost?"'
>
> (district nurse)

In this chapter I have examined one aspect of the nurses' questionnaire comments written over three years and, to a lesser extent, nurses' contribution to staff meetings held during the same period. It has also been possible to argue that many nurses negotiated a subjectivity that was forged out of conflicting discourses of caring and exploitation within their employing organisations. The result of this was a position aligned with self-sacrifice. The exercise of individual judgement at the site of caring might have been a point of resistance to managerial power but in many instances nurses described being frustrated in their exercise of judgement by the constraints of time. This was an uneasy position as it appeared to deny both power and, often, satisfaction, particularly as not only the financial but a wider realm of more abstract activity including the administrative and possibly the intellectual, were set up in opposition to 'practical caring'.

At the beginning of the chapter I announced that I would try to resist the temptation to write about nurses and managers in the ways that they spoke about each other – and themselves – because this would be to risk picturing identity as homogenous and stable. I am not sure how far I have succeeded. My intention has been to demonstrate that identity can be viewed as something that is achieved, in the context of discourse, rather than as an innate attribute. In Chapter 9 I will develop this thinking and explore what the outcomes of this investigation might mean both for the organisation of health services and for the research process.

9 Beyond oppression and profession

In this, the final chapter, I wish to reflect on whether my exploration of the texts of nurses and managers, and the literature I have looked at, enables us to think in new ways about:

- profession and power
- organisation(s) and power
- subjectivity/identity
- the project of inquiry

PROFESSION AND POWER

> The sociology of health and illness has defined itself, at least in part, through its illustrations of the darker side to caring relationships. The healers are exposed as manipulative and/or oppressive characters, quick to make judgmental and moral evaluations of their patients, or as agents of a deterministic social or political system.
>
> (Fox 1993: 70)

Fox's purpose here is to make some of sociology's modernist tendencies clear. One of these is undoubtedly its homogenising impulse; the sociology of health and illness appears, even in Fox's meticulous critique, as almost synonymous with medical sociology. Although nurses and others are included in its scrutiny – the quotation above could be applied to nursing – it would be unhelpful to see professionalism, or claims to some special privileged position, as achieved in the same way by different professional groups. The sociology of health and healing 'has been defined (and privileged) as the positive, empowering discipline – on the side of the oppressed and vulnerable' (ibid.: 71). But with nursing we have an ambiguous group that is both a profession, engaging in the 'darker' practices of professional life, and at the same time understanding *itself* as an oppressed group. In other ways, even within each of nursing's own groupings (health visitors, district nurses, school nurses) there are different projects under way. I have presented here one such project given voice in the comments of nurses involved in this study. Its privileging of the language of caring and its downgrading of the abstract should not be understood as representing a more generalised nursing characteristic, although the expression of caring is a major nursing theme. As others have shown, and I will be discussing this later in this chapter (see p. 164), managerialism has been taken up by a great many nurses, whether strategically by those in authoritative positions or less consciously by those positioned differently and I have detailed in Chapter 4 some of the nursing profession's efforts to maintain power. I am uncertain of the status of the project expressed by nurses in this study. It may represent the dying voice of a fading group or it may characterise a more robust position of a significant, but nevertheless unsanctioned nursing subgroup. It is unlikely to become an endorsed professional project, I would suggest, because of its self-conscious opposition to things nonphysical including education, its stance of disempowerment and its Luddite tendencies. However, its very negativity, lack of both political finesse and effectiveness and its failure to obey ascendant rules of rationality lend this project an admirable freedom of concept and argument. The nurses whose words I have assembled can voice unease, powerlessness, a sense of contradiction and anger in a way that more 'rational' operators who have more to lose in terms of credibility, power, position and influence can rarely achieve.

In what ways can a discourse of caring be understood as a project of power/knowledge and control? To begin to address such a question, Fox applies the psychoanalytic frameworks first of Jacques Lacan (1980) and then of Deleuze and Guattari (1984) to Talcott Parsons's well-known notion of the sick role and its repetitions of familial relations. Parsons considered that in many ways the sick person repeated aspects of a child's role in dependency and an expectation of care by stronger individuals (Parsons and Fox 1952). According to one of Fox's readings of Parsons, the part played by the doctor in sickness is to mediate the sick person's desire to return to a pre-oedipal stage of development, to give permission for the expression of such desires but eventually, by means of a retreat into professionalism, to discipline the patient's desires so that they begin to relinquish such a role. Working from the triadic relationship posited by Freud and developed by Lacan of 'Mother – Father – Ego', Fox suggests that the doctor in Parsons's account becomes identified not with the mother but with the 'Name of the Father'. Lacan claimed that in early stages of development as the child develops a new awareness of the presence of the father, it realises, unconsciously, that it cannot be its parent's lover and that it must give up its close bonds to its mother's body. This teaches the child, also unconsciously, the painful lessons of sexual difference, exclusion and absence. The child learns these lessons at the same time as it develops language and the two processes become inextricably linked, even identical. The child learns that language, or a signifier, presupposes the absence of the object it signifies, that language stands in for, or defers to, objects, substituting itself for possession of the object itself. The Name of the Father becomes associated with the realm of the symbolic, with a symbol of lack and a desire that is never fulfilled.

How does the nurse fit into this scheme? Parsons suggested that 'mother, father, therapist figure may be said to vary over a continuous range; with the mother giving the highest level of permissiveness and support; the physician, the greatest incentive to acceptance of discipline' (Parsons and Fox 1952: 42).

> The professionalism of the relationship is the means by which the association is made not with the Mother, satisfier of need, but with the Father, symbol of lack, which desire will seek to fill, but which is destined for ever to be unrequited.
>
> (Fox 1993: 82)

It is tempting but probably unhelpful to locate the nurse somewhere between 'mother' and 'physician' on the grounds of the nurse's (usual) gender and lesser authority (to legally authorise sickness) compared to the doctor. Fox argues that it will become second nature for the professional to use 'the dependency of the patient or other staff to assure authority' (ibid.: 83). It is uncertain how far the nurses involved in this study derived authority from their contact with patients; it is clearer that their identity, or aspects of it, rested upon their relationship to their patients. This is *possibly* a more benign version of the identity work that Fox describes the surgeon, Mr D, as being involved in: 'The patient . . . becomes a *repetition*, another in a long line of success stories. His subjectivity is territorialised within a framework which is discursively constituted in Mr D's desire to be a surgeon' (ibid.: 86; original emphasis)

Fox takes the possibilities for professional/patient relations into uncharted territory, guided by Deleuze and Guattari's notions of desire. I will not follow here but will only see how far his reflections on notions of the wounded healer can be applied to the nurses in this study.

In his book *The Wound and the Doctor* psychiatrist Bennet suggested that in history a dual attribute has often been attached to the healer, that of being him- or herself wounded and capable of healing (Bennet 1987). The healer has, through his or her experience, learned to relate to the wound creatively, so that through this creativity, others can be healed. The healer's mixture of weakness and strength, of 'competent doctor' and 'frightened patient', is said to be present in everyone. In Western health care, however, the professional carer has come to suppress the fear, helplessness and desire for care of their 'patient' side and so blocked the potential for self-healing present within all sick people. Deleuze and Guattari guide Fox to suggest that the 'helplessness and fear' of the patient side can better be understood more positively, as openness, trust and sharing and that self-healing is possible if the 'patient' resists the oedipal discourses of dependency constituted by professional care. It is hard to go far beyond conjecture when trying to understand how far the nurses in this study can be understood as 'wounded healers' who either accept or suppress their own fear. They certainly link their own suffering at being treated inhumanely by their organisations to (what they see as) the suffering of patients who face reduced services and a society that is increasingly uncaring. Both patient and nurse, they assert, are united in being victims of managerial self-interest and modern financial stringency. This anger seems at times to add impetus to their caring motivation, but I would hesitate to think of it as 'relating to the wound creatively'. Bennet saw the Western doctor typically as dominating in knowledge and power and forcing the patient into a supine position. The nurses in this study did not present themselves in this way but did present a strong dualism between the patient who *needed* caring and the nurse who was present and 'called' to meet these needs. Some talked of patient 'empowerment' and of encouraging self-sufficiency but these tended to be nurses in middle-management positions accounting for the need to 'rationalise' service delivery. The study's more typical nurses were dependent on the (perceived) dependency of those they cared for, for the performance of their identity as carers. Perhaps the identity of this group of nurses, and others like them, is at stake in the struggle over who is sanctioned to identify 'need'; the clinician faced with the distressed individual or those whose responsibility it is to account for services at an organisational level. (Of course, there are more than two 'groups' present in the health care arena.) It seemed that middle managers were being drawn into a new space by an 'unarguable' rationality created by financial constraint, New Right policy and the rise of technological surveillance, but felt unease and anxiety at the unintended consequences of such accounting procedures.

ORGANISATION(S) AND POWER: MANIFESTATIONS OF MODERNITY

The managers set out a new start for their organisations, or rather drew upon such a notion for their persuasion and part of their self-presentation. This involved an emphasis on rational approaches, on the techniques of measurement as well as on innovation. Managers frequently contrasted this new rationalism with the traditionalism and apparent irrationality of many within the nursing and medical workforce. They tended to describe nurses in terms of unconsidered and frenetic activity, like the 'headless chickens' referred to by one nurse executive, or as individually and collectively tradition-bound and lacking the confidence, training and imagination to innovate, take risks and adjust their activities to maximise effectiveness. Exceptions to this rule were the new breed of what one chief executive described as 'technocrats' who were said to be keen to embrace not only innovation but general management.

Even though the majority of managers involved in this study were women, so that it is not possible to present a simple picture of management as patriarchy in a predominantly female environment, any understanding that did not give attention to the gendering of the situation would be incomplete. Many feminists have seen the Enlightenment project as a male one and some of their critiques could equally well be applied to the managerial project in the present research. Hartsock sees the Enlightenment as a colonising endeavour, one in which the European conquests of the eighteenth and nineteenth centuries offer a parallel to phallocentric imperialism in which men devised a 'way of dividing up the world that puts an omnipotent subject at the centre and constructs marginal Others as sets of negative qualities . . . the colonised emerges as the image of everything the coloniser is not' (Hartsock 1990: 160, 161). Dorothy Smith argues that women have been assigned the kind of work that men did not want to do and in this sense 'women's work' relieves men of a range of activities such as taking care of their bodies (and, in this study, perhaps, the bodies of others) which allows them to consider as real only the realm of the abstract and the mental. 'Women's work' then becomes understood not as a consciously chosen activity but as natural, instinctual labour (Smith 1974). Such talk about nursing, and the supposed threat to its caring (and instinctual) character by its increasingly academic preparation, is still commonplace (Lawson 1996; Allen 1997).

Patriarchal beliefs have characterised women as bearers of tradition and men as bearers of modernity since the eighteenth century, if not before. For example, in the context of midwifery and obstetrics the forceps used by doctors in the delivery of babies reinforced this image of men by 'linking them with innovative techniques' (Jordanova 1989: 33). Although it would be dangerous to insist on too close, too deterministic an application of these theories to the present study, it could be argued, as does Davies in her account of bureaucracy as a gendered phenomenon (Davies 1995), that to the extent that a management perspective involves a progressive shift from the particular to the general and acontextual, it represents the ascendancy of a view of the world that has been associated with men. From this understanding, female managers have been enrolled by an inherently male system. Their characterisations of the female workforce as overly influenced by the particularity of their personal encounters in caring would be evidence for this claim. However, this view has problems. It essentialises gender and tends to underestimate the way in which subject positions are negotiated and to assume that it is impossible for women in 'male' positions to subvert the values and practices of that system. The various examples of 'split subjectivity' within the managers' texts in this study appeared to offer examples of attempts at such a subversion, although the complexity of self-presentation makes it hard to come to firm conclusions about such passages.

Modernity, surveillance and organisation

A picture of modern society as an increasingly 'disciplinary' society is now well developed. Surveillance has been given a place as an integral technology of this 'disciplinary' work and seen as an embodiment of the Enlightenment quest to dispel the areas of darkness in humanity and make all things knowable through the formalised procedures of observation, recording, measurement; the 'subjection through illumination' referred to by Foucault (1980a: 154). The first step in the creation of such a disciplinary society is the introduction of surveillance apparatus that can bring about continuous visibility or its ever present possibility which, it is expected, will lead to the most efficient form of control, self-regulation.

In the texts of the managers these organisational apparatuses appeared to take three forms; first, the nurturing among field workers of a sense of the solemn seriousness of regular self-disclosure. This took the form of attempting to forge links within the minds of field staff between certain ideas: the meticulous recording of daily activity, the numerical nature of contractual arrangements with purchasing organisations, and the possibility of losing income and staff posts should target activity levels not be reached. Second, the arrangement of people in space to facilitate surveillance was attempted by team formation and new levels of hierarchy involving team leaders, leaders of team leaders and intensified professional supervision. Community nursing sisters, once a relatively autonomous mass of foot soldiers, now reduced in number, were increasingly expected to take on a supervisory role over lesser qualified and unqualified workers and to be constantly answerable to managers for their professional decisions. Third, appealing to finance as a given and to attractive notions of professional autonomy and even patient empowerment enabled managers to adopt a rhetoric of offering freedom of choice to field staff while actually exercising detailed and overarching control. Many managers offered as evidence of the fairness and acceptability of changes in skill-mix the fact that the drive for more hours and less skills came from field staff themselves. This is hardly surprising and can be seen as capitalising on staff's urgent sense of the overwhelming need of their clients. The 'devolving' of budgets to local or even individual level can be understood as an exploitation of Peters and Waterman's advice that a sense of even small control increases performance greatly (Peters and Waterman 1982). Using all these techniques, supported by the use of computer recording and telecommunications, the eighteenth-century practices of enclosure, such as the army camp, the school and the hospital, were extended unimaginably.

Organisation, authority and the art of persuasion

This research has pictured the managers as 'wily rhetorician[s]' exercising a 'will to persuade'. Ricoeur reminds us that metaphor 'redescribes' reality (Ricoeur 1986: 22) and that skill at rhetoric has been seen as affording its user formidable power to 'manipulate words apart from things, and to manipulate men by manipulating words' (ibid.: 11). Organisational writers urge managers to accumulate such skills although they generally erase the moral and political from their exhortations. Peters and Waterman advocate attention to the 'cultural' aspect of organisational life and a host of other management writers emphasise the crucial importance of the manager's initial target for organisational change being the ideas of the workforce, rather than its roles and structures (Van de Ven 1980; Spurgeon and Barwell 1991). This echoes Foucault's descriptions of the increasingly subtle nature of discipline exercised over populations during the eighteenth and nineteenth centuries (Foucault 1977). Gahmberg describes 'metaphor management' as part of the successful manager's 'creation of a meaningful context for the organisational members' (Gahmberg 1990).

Swales and Rogers argue that management literature has consistently recognised the importance of language in business affairs and that one key, tangible sign of change within an organisation is that its language is changing. Through language 'meaning is created and action becomes possible' (Swales and Rogers 1995: 224).

MacIntyre addresses the notion of manipulation when considering the managerial claims to moral neutrality and effectiveness which he considers central to the way that contemporary managers present themselves. He first demonstrates that anyone wishing to persuade another to carry out a particular course of action has two different approaches at their disposal. The first is the use of personal criteria where the hearer's decision to act depends upon a range of personal and contextual factors: 'do this because I wish it'. The second, which MacIntyre argues is characteristic of our culture and times, involves the speaker's appeal to purportedly impersonal, rational criteria: 'do this because it is your duty' or 'do this because it would give pleasure to a number of people'. The second form of persuasion can be considered manipulative persuasion because, in an age where there are no agreed and unassailable criteria for moral action, such appeals confer an objectivity on utterances that are no more than expressions of their speaker's own preference (MacIntyre 1985). MacIntyre links claims for managerial effectiveness to those of moral neutrality by suggesting that effectiveness is an unavoidably moral conception because it is 'inseparable from a mode of human existence in which the contrivance of means is in central part the manipulation of human beings into compliant patterns of behaviour' (ibid.: 74). Claims to effectiveness, and hence authority, amount to little more than a moral fiction, he argues, because there is no body of knowledge upon which managers can draw by means of which organisations and social structures can be shaped. Both of these claims, to the existence of a domain of moral neutrality and to effectiveness through access to a range of law-like generalisations, MacIntyre suggests:

> mirror claims made by the natural sciences; and it is not surprising that expressions such as 'management science' should be coined. The manager's claim to moral neutrality, which is itself an important part of the way the manager presents himself and functions in the social and moral world, is thus parallel to the claims to moral neutrality made by many physical scientists.
>
> (ibid.: 77)

The extent to which the managers in this study spoke about their decisions and actions in terms of moral neutrality is debatable. (The nursing field staff clearly presented their own work in morally committed terms.) At points in the text, the managers referred to the generalised operation of financial principles, 'maximising returns on our investments' (chief executive, Optimist Community Health Trust), to the workings of market forces, to the making of decisions based on impersonal criteria such as the redundancies of medical officers in Pragmatic Community Health Services, and to abstaining from overt political comment (chief executive, Pragmatic Community Health Services). Yet the whole rhetorical context appears to be one of a moral commitment to the specific activity of providing health care services. Defining 'core business', value and mission statements, the subject position of acting in the public interest and the revolutionary talk of many managers to challenge the domination of both medicine and the acute hospitals' monopolisation of resources, were all presented as moral acts. It could be that in the context of this research, with the nursing focus of the study, managers chose to inhabit the subjectivity of the high ethical tone and that in other contexts other emphases would have been brought to the fore to serve different purposes. It could be that the managers' claim to be *more effective than clinicians* in organising health care services rests on a firm assertion of the efficacy of those managerial techniques that differentiate them from clinicians. This was, after all, the central claim of the Griffiths report which has acted as the starting-point for so many significant changes to the UK health service since its appearance.

A final speculation on the current ascendancy of the rationality of measurement is prompted both by MacIntyre's insights into the masquerade of managerial control and by the thoughts of Lyotard on the commercialisation of modern art. In *The Postmodern Condition*, Lyotard argued that the era of the metanarrative is over, in terms of science, culture and the arts. Eclecticism is the defining characteristic of contemporary culture. However, eclecticism in the realm of art presents a problem to those seeking to make evaluative decisions about alternatives. One response has been to evaluate against a single criteria, that of financial yield:

> Artists, gallery owners, critics, and public wallow together in the 'anything goes'.. [but].. in the absence of aesthetic criteria, it remains possible and useful to assess the value of works of art according to the profits they yield.
> (Lyotard 1979: 76)

It could be argued that in developed Western societies, health care presents a similar problem. We are faced with an ever increasing range of possible interventions and with attempts to reduce expenditure but are faced at the same time with the loss of faith in an overarching medical authority. There are now a multiplicity of voices competing for a say on ever more complex health care decisions. The strategy of governments has lain in being seen to be making decisions on the basis of some form of rational criteria. '[O]bjectivist discourses are not just the territory of intellectuals and academics,' notes Sandra Harding, 'they are the official dogma of the age' (Harding 1990: 88). The health needs assessment that, in theory, forms the basis of the purchasing that was intended to drive the UK internal market (Ham 1991) and the Labour government's Health Improvement Programmes (Department of Health 1997), are such attempts. The Oregon experiment in the United States (Klevit *et al.* 1991), in which the local population were given an opportunity to contribute to decisions about which health care procedures were funded in that state, produced a troubling outcome which involved the vetoing of the scheme by President George Bush in 1992 (McBride 1992). In the absence of a more convincing moral consensus, the form of rationality adopted by governments has been utilitarian. If managers at the local level can direct their efforts towards the measurement, control and efficient distribution of health care inputs, they might maintain something close to the masquerade of potency that MacIntyre argues masks a fundamental powerlessness within corporations and governments (MacIntyre 1985).

SUBJECTIVITY/IDENTITY: COLONISATION RECONSIDERED

It is all too easy to oppose the arguments of the managers and nurses in the same dualistic terms in which they take up and sometimes parody each other's arguments to use them for their own purposes. The success of the managers' project and the achievement of their identity depends, in part, upon how well they can interpret clinicians as irrational, self-seeking, financially profligate and therefore in need of managerial discipline. Clinicians, for their part, attempt to stand between the government or managers and public support by pointing to the contradiction between managers' talk of efficiency and their expansion in numbers and cost, or by casting them as limited, even tainted, by their association with industry and commerce, excluded from the intimacy, humanity and immense power of the clinician's relationship with the patient. (The incoming UK Labour government in 1997 clearly shared the first view and their initial White Paper on the NHS featured the project of cutting down on bureaucracy. The outgoing Conservatives had begun to address this after having presided over a massive increase in managerial numbers.) It is hard to resist being drawn onto this dualistic ground and use it to dramatic and persuasive effect. However, the power and effect of the dualism that both groups draw upon depends on ambient cultural dualisms, like that between rationality and irrationality. Though it is impossible to do away with these dualisms altogether, it is feasible to destabilise them and to show, in this instance, how these two groups depend on them to further their own projects and even rely upon some essential aspect of the qualities they reject as (belonging to the) other.

The image of the European conquest of the Iroquois conjured up at the beginning of Chapter 1 carried with it a certain simplicity and a fatalism, an assumption that power is always oppressive and imposed on passive subjects. Yet post-structuralist accounts of the operation of power have made a more careful analysis possible and it is time to consider some of these in relation to the question of nursing and managerialism. Lupton poses certain key questions in her exploration of the character of 'critical discourse analysis':

 . . . how do individuals take up, negotiate, or resist discourse and how is
resistance generated and sustained? What are the constraints to taking up

subject positions? How are the individuals interpellated, or 'hailed' by discourses – how do they recognise themselves within?

(Lupton 1995: 302)

For senior managers, it appeared that the new discourse of managerialism addressed them as individuals who could exercise an unprecedented control over their destiny. The way that involvement in the reforms was constituted by the Conservative government as a voluntary action (management teams could 'express interest' and then apply to become involved) emphasised the point that acceptance of the reforms, their language and their ethos, was an empowering autonomous decision. During the period before the reforms and in their early days, according to one speaker, management teams who were expressing an interest or who accepted the invitation to participate received a great deal of suggestion from 'politicians' that they were innovators in a 'brave new world' (nurse executive, Optimist Community Health Trust), reinforcing and extending the notion of autonomy. Also, perhaps, involvement in what the same manager termed the Trust 'movement', might involve newly energised career opportunities. One nurse executive involved in the study became chief executive shortly after the research finished. If these offers were not sufficient attractions to prospective participants, a suspicion that in the future the terms of participation would not afford similar advantages and similar control, provided the last persuasion. Therefore the reforms also addressed individuals as pragmatists.

For managers with a clinical background, the appeal of the reforms was perhaps more complex than for those from administrative and managerial origins. General management, with which nurse executives had already evidently come to terms, and now the market reforms, held an explicit challenge to health professionals that might appear problematic. Clinicians had to adopt particular discursive manoeuvres in order to accommodate its demands. One apparently successful way of achieving this was by an appeal to notions of social justice and to 'acting in the public's best interests'. Any challenge to the professions was pictured as a restoration of the true service ethos to professionals who had become self-serving and complacent. However, as I have previously argued, claims that 'everything is done with the client's needs in perspective first, and the professional needs following up the rear' (nurse executive, Pragmatic Community Health Services) may demonstrate little more than the ideological power of rhetoric and subjectivity in an environment where managers, through financial constraint, had devised a 'core service' of minimal interventions.

Another aspect of 'acting in the public's best interest' took the form of utilitarianism, an equitable dispersion of the scarce resource of community nursing health care, rationally planned and consciously targeted at those objectively identified as most in need. Paradoxically, and perhaps as an example of the fluid nature of subjectivity, the nurse executives also expressed strong desires to enhance the influence and standing of professional nursing, to save it from becoming 'the handmaiden of all the other professions' (nurse executive, Optimist Community Health Trust) or so that they might see nursing 'come to the forefront' (nurse executive, Pragmatic Community Health Services). They cited the very reforms that had been widely heralded and understood as being introduced to curb professional power as mechanisms for achieving this vision. As Lupton argues:

> It is difficult to continue to argue that individuals share fixed concerns and membership of defined social groups. An individual who has a certain political allegiance at one moment may have a different, conflicting allegiance at another.
>
> (Lupton 1995: 302)

Those sceptical managers, who occupied positions lower in the management hierarchies of the organisations under study and were exclusively from nursing backgrounds, tended to characterise themselves as reluctant followers with little, if any, opportunity to take up power and control. If the reforms had hailed them as autonomous individuals, the call had fallen on deaf ears. Nevertheless, even this group appeared to find certain aspects of the changes unchallengeable, most notably those 'housekeeping' aspects, as Mrs Thatcher would say, which were concerned with using resources more self-consciously. At moments, they constructed the experience of nurses having less time for their clients in terms of a discourse of self-help, client-empowerment and avoidance of the worst dependency-generating effects of welfare state provision, 'the nanny state' (local manager, Pragmatic Community Health Services). Theirs appeared to be an uncomfortable position which frequently involved struggling for words during the interviews because the vocabulary they wanted was undeveloped, apparently outmoded or outlawed in their organisations. Half of the sceptics were relatively close to retirement and thus opportunities for a revitalised management career on the crest of the NHS reforms were less available. They tended to draw upon their length of service with the NHS to characterise their resistance to the changes by describing themselves as 'old-fashioned' (local manager, Pragmatic Community Health Services). The pointed irony of such a posture allowed them to create a space within which they could set up an opposition between the past and present in terms of traditional, human values on the one hand, and a new bureaucracy and efficiency on the other. They did this in a way that allowed them to express a sense of alienation from certain of those values.

I have already described some of the ways that the nursing workforce attempted to resist a managerial discourse of efficiency and rationality, by characterising itself as involved in a self-sacrificial moral activity. Nurses had to reconcile the discourses of caring with those of exploitation and disempowerment. The discursive tactic adopted to align these two positions was that of the personal sacrifice. In this sense, the application of managerial power gave rise to this particular sense of subjectivity. However, within this apparently highly constrained situation, they attempted to hold on to a sense of autonomy by linking their professional judgement with their sense of moral agency. A Nietzschean perspective, within which we could understand the rationality of managers as a manifestation of the 'will to power', might view the moral orientation and indignation of the nurses as a sign of their 'slave morality' (Nietzsche 1994).

Callon *et al.* (1986) and Latour (1987) have developed the notions of 'enrolment' and 'alignment of interests', to explain how a variety of social actors seek to achieve their purposes by aligning the interests of others with their own. Joanna Latimer has used these notions in a number of studies to provide a compelling explanation for nurses' and doctors' uptake of a managerial priority to maintain hospital throughput. In one ethnographic study (Latimer 1997a), clinicians call on notions of the 'acute' nature of their practice in order to figure certain elderly patients as 'social' rather than medical and hence misplaced in an acute project and in the acute hospital ward. They are 'bed-blockers' and their removal is legitimated on these grounds. Their continued presence threatens the convincing performance and the purity of the acute project. Managers, or others, whose overriding requirement may be to maintain cost-effective hospital throughput, can align clinicians to this purpose without overt disciplinary activity. She argues that:

> Nurses' practices can be understood ... as not simply functional or instrumental, moral or spiritual, but as expressive of identity. .... Nurses, to belong, perform in ways that help to make them visible as 'nurses', 'employees', 'professionals', 'colleagues', 'good' etc. In other words, nurses, as they practise, are doing 'identity-work' in multiple domains.
>
> (Latimer 1997b: 45)

Interestingly, while her work shows nurses to have taken up aspects of managerialism, it would be difficult to come to the same conclusion within this study. One possible reason for this difference may lie in the different settings in which the two investigations were carried out, an acute ward and Community Trusts. Again, while not wanting to simplify the 'identity-work' of nurses involved in this study, there was little evidence that they could wholeheartedly adopt identities as employee or organisational member. The notions of enrolment and translation of interests, however, do provide powerful explanations for managers' uptake of the reforms.

Yet to what extent and in what ways did the nurses take up the 'official' discourses of their professional leaders and organisations, some of which have been outlined in Chapter 4? In what sense were they having to reconcile these and dominant discourses within their organisations? As we have seen in Chapter 4, nursing leaders have made efforts to ensure that they shape and reshape professional discourse in a way that maximises its contemporary credibility so that at the time of writing, for example, talk of nursing from its leaders is in terms of evidence-based practice, the identification of measurable outcomes, improving of the educational basis of its practitioners and contributing unique insights to clinical governance. These are all linked to, or legitimated by, the notion of solidarity with the patient and recipient of care. At the height of the market reforms, issues of 'marketing your services' were being widely discussed and sometimes promoted in nursing's popular journals (Edwards 1994). However, it was notable that the nurses who were involved in this study did not appear to draw upon these discourses and in fact many expressed distance from the values they embodied.

There is perhaps no way of knowing why these 'official' discourses appeared to hold little relevance for the nurses involved in this study. It seems that nurses tended to site their subjectivity in the 'needs-based/caring-as-duty' moral framework, or something close to it, that at least one nursing leader has described as 'definitely passé' (Kitson 1993). This characterisation of nursing appears to owe much to Nightingale (Mason 1991) and is said, for example by Menzies, to have had a detrimental impact on nurses' emotional life (Menzies 1960), although more recently the centrality of caring and its ethical value have been re-emphasised by Leininger (1978) and Watson (1985). Nevertheless, the point remains that those more contemporary discourses of effectiveness and marketability were virtually nonexistent within the comments of the nurses. It may be that, although it could be advantageous for nurses to take them up, these discourses had failed to shape the sense of self or the discourse of the main part of community nurses for some intrinsic reason, possibly because they clashed with a more powerful discourse already established. It may be that, merely given time, these discourses will be adopted and that their absence from the talk of nurses in this study does not indicate resistance to them. Or it may be that the nurses who participated in this study do indeed resist these discourses while a great many others have accepted them and the participants represent a particular voice, one that may possibly grow quieter over future years. Indeed, the only notable change over the course of this study to the character of the nurses' contributions was a sharp decline in comments expressing strong hostility to management and the reforms between the first and successive years.

I now return to issues concerning reflection on research methodology.

THE PROJECT OF INQUIRY

The radically sceptical nature of a postmodern approach to inquiry can lead to a particular kind of unease. This project may present intellectual challenges and furnish a sense of satisfaction that it might provide a convincing account of certain phenomena within UK health care that could be extended to an increasing range of public affairs in Western societies. However, on the one hand, claims to an authoritative explanation that might form a basis for policy formation or, on the other, involvement in an emancipatory project for nursing do not sit easily with such work. Postmodernism has been criticised as failing on both these grounds, although often its critics such as Taylor-Gooby (1994) appear to fall back on Enlightenment language and the status quo as an alternative, and those who critique the lack of emancipatory purchase of some of its work can hardly avoid implicitly privileging the authority of the researcher or the position and view of a particular group which is deemed marginal. On the second point, my understanding of subjectivity involves a sense that the marginality of any group is largely contextual. The nursing profession, for example, has often been presented as marginal to the immense political strong-hold of mainstream scientific medicine yet, from a reading of its leaders' work, it is possible to see it as a similar power elite with aspirations to increase that power. Later in this chapter (see pp. 170–174) I will discuss and argue a case against many of these criticisms of postmodernism's apparent failure to provide a basis for policy or action.

As this research has proceeded, any sense of an authority for it linked to a method or approach that rests upon an epistemological grounding, has become progressively more antithetical. This process started with the impact of Rorty's description of inquiry as a recontextualising of beliefs, rather than as representa-tion, and with his refusal to differentiate interpretation from explanation, with the latter's appeals to reason (Rorty 1991b). The process proceeded through Foucault's identification of the inhibiting effect of totalising theories (Foucault 1980b) and the danger of changing one discursive identity for another and in the process creating new oppressions.

The final (so far) part of this movement has involved taking up deconstruc-tion's rejection of the traditional distinction between the literary text and the critical work (de Man 1979) and applying that to the research endeavour. Just as deconstruction acknowledges that the critical enterprise itself is bound to use the same persuasive techniques as the works it attempts to unravel, this research claims no privileged access to truth about the texts it analyses and attempts to deconstruct. This work is ultimately rhetorical, as is the case, I would argue, for inquiry that does claim access to a metaphysical grounding, whether that grounding be located in scientific methodology or in the privilege of direct experience or insight. Nevertheless, I would insist that this work has its own rigour and structure and is not arbitrary. In discussing the influence of deconstruction with its discovery of the rhetorical nature of philosophical arguments, Norris suggests that literary works could be understood as 'less deluded than the discourse of philosophy, precisely because they implicitly acknowledge and exploit their own rhetorical status' (Norris 1991: 21). As Rorty acknowledges, even though there may be no noncircular justification for doing what we do, this does not prevent us from arguing our case with passion (Rorty 1991b).

In one reflection upon some of these issues as they relate to research in nursing, Parsons discusses the issues in terms of two 'crises' that postmodernism might be seen to precipitate for research methodology: crises of legitimation and representation and modern conceptions of knowledge (Parsons 1995). This picture of knowledge involves unproblematic understandings of the self, the object of knowledge, the relationship between the two and the language with which we might designate and describe these objects. Parsons details how notions of accuracy or authenticity of account stem from a privileging of the original context of the research participants' words and activities. A significant erosion of this notion took place with the understanding of language as an ideological production. If ideology presupposes an alternative, i.e. an authentic way of understanding the world, postmodernism has questioned even this, leading the inquirer into social situations with no solid ground upon which to base their project. Researchers have adopted a number of strategies to avoid this dilemma. These have tended to be pragmatic and procedural rather than philosophical and included the featuring of multiple voices in the research report and the reflexive inclusion of the researcher who adds 'his or her own voice to the data'. However, these approaches have problems. First, because they appear to be based upon a static and unified conception of the self, that the researcher, like the groups and interests presented, do each have a unitary 'voice' and second, because there is a silence about the overarching, invisible and organising 'self' of the researcher who carefully blends and balances a range of different views including their own. A doubled subjectivity is already present in the description of the researcher 'adding their voice to the data'.

This same static and unitary view of the self, I suggest, lies behind some unresolved problems with Parsons's argument, that is, the designation of 'the oppressed' and the privileging of the experience of the professional nurse. There is a twin assumption here. First, that a more real or authentic self lies beneath the 'layers of social guises' that she sees illness as stripping away and that this process somehow levels 'oppressed and oppressor alike' who are seen as two distinct groups rather than fluid and contextual designations and subjectivities. Second, that even if there is this authentic world of, in the words of Shakespeare's King Lear, the 'unaccommodated man', professional nurses have a unique access to it that is denied to 'the sociologist, anthropologist, political scientist, philosopher, economist or other social researcher'. Again there is the assertion that people involved in any of these disciplines are confined by their professional roles and are condemned to observe and interact with the 'theatrical selves' of others.

A final methodological point of interest in Parsons's argument concerns the account of attempts to confer validity upon qualitative research studies by the presentation of study findings to those involved in the field work for their ratification of the researcher's interpretation. This has become a widespread practice (Webb 1993; Denzin and Lincoln 1994; Seibold *et al.* 1994; Morse and Field 1996). While the dangers of researchers asserting their own understanding of events and situations over and above those of the actors involved in the research and the use of notions such as 'false consciousness' to support this have been thoroughly discussed (Lather 1986, 1991), I would argue that there is a certain power imbalance inherent in the presentation of any version of words and events by an organising presenter. Perhaps it is a lingering positivism that is problematic, with its suggestion that the research report claims a particular authority of technique or objectivity, that it offers a 'reality' to which the subjects of research as victims of ideology may not have access. There lurks also, perhaps, what Derrida refers to as the privileging of presence in terms of conscious intention as the ultimate arbiter of meaning.

In the present work I answer these issues in the following way. First, the power structures that influence and shape language, argumentation and possibilities for identity are not always, or even usually, a matter of conscious intention but nevertheless perform certain functions. Second, to the extent that we have an interest in and maintain power from the subject positions we adopt, we are likely to respond in particular ways to those who articulate this process, question it or point to some troublesome contradictions. The characteristic of dialogue between researcher and researched may well be a potentially unending rhetorical agonistics rather than a process of verification by adjustment and consensus.

Criticism and critique of postmodernism

Taylor-Gooby: Postmodernism has undermined policy critique

Taylor-Gooby looks at what he sees as the unhelpful influence of postmodernism on the development of social policy. He argues first that postmodernism's refusal to accept any universal explanations or bases for thought and action means that it can provide no strong or unified critique of the global influence of economic liberalism which he describes as the 'nearest approximation to a universal theme in world affairs' (Taylor-Gooby 1994: 388). In fact, he argues, postmodernism's emphasis on plurality and the local, and its questioning of the role of the nation-state actively plays into the individualism inherent in New Right market liberalism. Like others, his critique is that postmodernism is an essentially nihilistic distraction:

> If postmodernism is suggesting that the intellectual trajectory of the modern state has arrived at a position where different values and interests with their supporting baggage of theory are seen to be of equal validity, and if the possibility of developing a method to choose between competing claims is abandoned, the approach is vulnerable to criticism: if nothing can be said with any certainty, it is perhaps better to say nothing.
>
> (ibid.: 393)

However, it emerges that Taylor-Gooby tends to focus on the periodising 'cultural description' postmodernism of Lyotard and others rather than post-modernism's highly effective philosophical critiques of modernity. This leads to confusion between talk of the 'universality' of social and political problems following in the wake of New Right policy with postmodernism's critiques of the 'universality' and totalitarian effects of the authority of reason. It is not so much that 'nothing can be said with any certainty' but that the basis of certainty is ultimately contextual. Postmodernism offers critics of social policy the opportunity to pinprick policy-makers' claims to universality and to reinter-pret their rhetoric-masquerading-as-logic, but they are inevitably drawn into the same ambivalent space as those they critique. Taylor-Gooby is right to cite Giddens's arguments that we live in a time, not of postmodernity, but of 'high modernity' (Giddens 1992) where the power of national governments and industrial capitalism to control and penetrate are as strong as ever, but he and other critics fail to make clear and question the basis of their own commitment to justice and to emancipation from social and political oppression. Taylor-Gooby cannot but adopt an unquestioned Enlightenment language in defence of his position in his supposition that '[s]ocial policy research is concerned to generate high quality objective knowledge that can be deployed in social planning' (Taylor-Gooby 1994: 387).

Liberation from undecidability – the undecidability of liberation

In order to assess how far postmodernism can be incorporated into a Marxian emancipatory project, Kincheloe and McLaren attempt to draw a distinction between what they term *postmodernity* which they see as descriptions of a cultural situation and *postmodern theory* which they describe as antifoundationalist writing in philosophy and the social sciences. They go perhaps a step too far by drawing a further distinction within postmodern theory between the unhelpful 'ludic' strand ('see, e.g., Lyotard, Derrida, Baudrillard' they suggest in what looks like a careless moment of Francophobia) and oppositional or critical postmodernism, the latter having forged connections with 'those egalitarian impulses of modernism that contribute to an emancipatory democracy' (Kincheloe and McLaren 1994). Kincheloe and McLaren of course have a point that the logic of language has a social and political context (this understanding forms the basis of certain styles of discourse analysis) but it seems inaccurate to suggest that the three theorists they blame for such unhelpful influences would deny this. Ludic (playful, ludicrous perhaps) postmodernism is described as everything that its critical relative is not. It is free-floating, spectral, ungrounded, radically uncertain, textual; rather than weighty, having a normative foundation, materialist, associated with praxis and rooted in the 'real' social and historical. There is a clear contrast between the nonserious and the serious. They recommend that critical researchers should adopt a 'cautionary stance' towards this source of distraction. What is disconcerting about Kincheloe and McLaren's view, at least from the perspective of undecidability, is the epistemological confidence with which they argue their case. What they term a 'conversation' between postmodern undecidability and a critical praxis sounds more like a monologue: 'As it invokes its strategies for the emancipation of meaning, critical theory provides the postmodern critique with a normative foundation (i.e. a basis for distinguishing between oppressive and liberatory social relations)' (ibid.: 144).

Although there must be some shared ground between these two positions, the conclusion that these criticalists live in a simplified world where meaning can undergo one globalising 'liberation', where there are criteria at hand to distinguish between the oppressive and the liberatory is hard to resist. My conclusion about Kincheloe and McLaren's conversation or attempted synthesis is that while it is vital to understand the interplay between language and political ideology, in the final reckoning, their (perhaps optimistic view of) 'conversation' amounts to a colonisation where the class struggle and liberation from oppression are the essential elements of a totalising project to which every other activity must contribute.

One critic of critical theory has made a similar point, arguing that the critical project is ultimately inconsistent because it: 'require[s] an epistemological theory which can justify the claim that critical researchers are able to gain genuine knowledge of social reality rather than being deceived by appearances like everyone else' (Hammersley 1995: 30).

One attempt to formulate such a theory has been Marxism in which appeal is made to a Hegelian teleological metanarrative in which the unfolding of history is said to gradually reveal true knowledge. Although advocates of postmodernism and critical theorists are sometimes said to be working together on the same project, post-structuralists and postmodernists are among the strongest critics of critical theory because the former question the latter's attempts to ground critique:

> From the point of view of post structuralism and postmodernism, critical theory is not critical enough. It is regarded as relying on the Enlightenment assumption that the exercise of reason can produce demonstrable truths about how society should be organised and how change can be brought about.
>
> (Hammersley 1995: 34)

Nevertheless, Hammersley, like Taylor-Gooby, appears to base his own work upon the problematic maxim that 'fighting oppression is a good thing: that is almost a logical truth' (ibid.: 44).

Feminism/postmodernism/and/Foucault

Postmodernism has been debated by many feminists and many of the key issues have been presented in a useful landmark of collected essays (Nicholson 1990). It is interesting to look at the work of two of the contributors to that collection who come to different conclusions about the issue. The first is Nancy Hartsock. In a similar vein to Kincheloe and McLaren, she warns that 'postmodernism represents a dangerous approach for any marginalised group to adopt'. She goes on to ask the perceptive question:

> Why is it that just at the moment when so many of us who have been silenced begin to demand the right to name ourselves, to act as subjects rather than objects of history, that just then the concept of subjecthood becomes problematic?
>
> (Hartsock 1990: 163)

Hartsock's focus here is on Foucault. Drawing on the collection *Power/Knowledge. Selected Interviews, and Other Writings 1972–1977* (Foucault 1980a) she argues that in Foucault's analysis of power, in which individuals circulate among the threads of power, simultaneously undergoing and exercising power, structural inequalities like those concerning class or gender disappear. Hartsock argues that Foucault's net-like image of power carries the implication that everyone caught up in this net is in some way equal, possibly even actively participating in their own subordination. For Hartsock, Foucault does not say enough about the 'systematic domination of the many by the few'. Foucault fails also to give any basis for resistance, suggesting that if our resistance succeeded, we would in effect be exchanging one discursive identity for another and in doing so create new oppressions. This is less than useful for any group who wish not just to resist but to transform oppressive situations, and even, as Hartsock does, to construct a new society. It is hard to imagine Foucault rising to such a rallying cry.

What can usefully be taken from Foucault's analysis of power is this: that it is possible that the effects of power include the constitution of particular types of subjectivity and that subjectivity can be understood as multiple in the sense that the individual, in one particular subjectivity, can undergo oppression, while in another, can exercise domination. (This is perhaps too awkward a way of putting it.) The nurse, to take one example, can be understood as subject to the immense power exercised by managers, the medical establishment and male epistemology. Simultaneously she can be seen as implicated in professional domination over the patient or other health care workers, using many of the same technologies of power as other professional groups. This multiple subjectivity does not mean that Foucault's insights, his ascending analysis of power, are not available to those who wish to theorise their own experience of oppression. What it does mean is that no group is able to launch into the project of constructing a new society without, in some sense, creating their own structural oppressions. What Foucault offers is a critique that makes it possible for individuals or groups to investigate the ways in which they may be complicit in their own subordination. This awareness need not be paralysing but can temper and give sophistication to transformative work. The structural aspects of power relations such as gender, class or race need not disappear in a 'Foucauldian' analysis – they become partial, albeit powerful explanations. After Foucault 'the oppressed' cannot claim a privileged epistemology. Delegitimated and disqualified discourses may urgently need to be disinterred in order to destabilise oppressive regimes, but they are discourses all the same. 'Oppressed' groups may engage in consciousness-raising but should not claim to have 'liberated meaning' and 'sort[ed] out who we really are' as Hartsock suggests. Liberation, emancipation and consciousness-raising can be understood as the mounting of offensives on totalising regimes in order to contribute to redefining what counts as truth (i.e. legitimate discourse) in particular communities of practice. They cannot be understood as redefining a universal truth that dwells outside all discourses.

Linda Nicholson, in contrast, argues that it is possible to develop a kind of postmodern feminist theory that is 'both politically and philosophically preferable to feminist theory uninfluenced by postmodern concerns' (Nicholson 1992: 82). She argues this by suggesting that postmodernism is not in fact as radical or nihilistic as it is often made out and that it need not lead us into an enervating relativism as has sometimes been claimed. Key postmodernist writers, she says, have never abandoned the possibility of truth criteria immanent to the practices which generate them, nor even the possibility of 'cross-cultural tools of adjudication such as a commitment to dialogue or the law of non-contradiction'. For her, like Rorty, it is the aspects of a common tradition shared by different groups that enable the possibility of dialogue. Also Nicholson attempts to examine more closely postmodernism's supposed conflation of truth and power. The two may be associated but they are not identical, she says. A distinction is possible because there is such a thing as illegitimate power, that is, power exercised outside the rules of a given community's discursive practice. Neither is there anything necessarily contradictory about a postmodern theory, she argues, provided theory is understood not as a transcendental explanation 'from nowhere' but pragmatically as a tool that proves to be more or less useful for our purposes. In short, postmodernism does not constitute the absolute break with modernity that has sometimes been suggested. This would be to generalise the meaning of postmodernism so that, just like the theories of modernism, it becomes a position outside history.

Nicholson is perhaps too optimistic about the possibility for dialogue between different communities, too optimistic that legitimate power can be differentiated from illegitimate. It can be argued that truth regimes such as those associated with the institutions of science and more recently managerialism are not content to exist in liberal-minded peace alongside 'superstition' or 'tradition'. A look, for example, at the health service situation in many developed countries today, or at Western welfare more generally reveals how the political forces of the New Right and managerialism have powerfully and effectively redefined what counts as truth in these contexts. So in a sense, Nicholson's account can be seen as paying too little attention to broader social power inequalities while Kincheloe and McLaren's sees this as the only issue of importance.

Foxiness and feminisms

Patti Lather also grapples with these problems (Lather 1991). She makes her ultimate commitment to 'oppositional' theory and practice clear yet she takes the challenge posed by postmodernism seriously, enjoying, in the process, its disruptions. She regards claims that postmodernism is a new fashion in theoreticism which does not provide sufficient unequivocal ground from which either to recommend action or to act, as a 'blackmail to urgency'. This blackmail, in effect, insists that 'post-structuralism make clear its practicality before it has barely begun to develop' (ibid.: 9). Her epistemological theory, or the nearest she wishes to get to one, which might justify the claim that critical researchers are able to gain genuine knowledge of social reality rather than being deceived by appearances, draws upon a neo-Marxist notion of the proletariat's ability to 'see through' ideology because of their position in relation to it. However, her claim is not for the truth but for a troublesome vision that can destabilise discourse – unless the demystifying that she refers to in the quotation below represents an attempt to discover the 'real thing' through the mists of ideology. She draws upon Ebert (1988):

> If one is always situated in ideology, then the only way to demystify these ideological operations . . . is to occupy the interstices of contesting ideologies or to seek the disjunctures and opposing relations created within a single ideology by its own contradictions.
>
> (Lather 1991: 11)

Lather situates her own work at the margins of 'feminisms, Neo-Marxisms and poststructuralisms'. She feels that such a position sensitises her to some of the questions that postmodernism can pose for liberatory pedagogues:

> . . . tied to their version of truth and interpreting resistance as 'false consciousness', too often such pedagogies fail to probe the degree to which 'empowerment' is something done 'by' liberated pedagogues 'to' or 'for' the as-yet-unliberated, the 'other', the object upon which is directed the emancipatory actions. . . . In this post-Marxist space, the binaries that structure liberatory struggle implode from 'us versus them' and 'liberation' versus 'oppression' to a multi-centred discourse with differential access to power.
>
> (Lather 1991: 16, 25)

Ultimately, she advocates a pragmatic 'foxiness' and 'versatility' so that at a time such as this when the theoretical tide has turned away from essentialised categories, we might still use such categories as 'woman' as if they existed when it is strategically to our advantage and question them at other moments. Such a 'double' approach can avoid the elitism implicit in grand theorising which attempts or purports to speak for all women but which, to the extent that it originates from a particular group, leaves out certain others such as, for example, women of colour or differently abled women. The same observation can perhaps be made regarding the category of 'nurse' which might suppress the huge variety of paid and unpaid workers and allows a particular kind of professional to stand in their place.

Lather's analysis represents a useful and sophisticated response to postmodernism from a committed emancipator. Her own 'double' approach, her conscious split-subjectivity, is consistent with her post-structuralist understanding of power, oppression and identity. She avoids privileging the emancipatory project as a 'liberation of meaning', a freeing from ideology into truth, while at the same time not relinquishing transformatory ambitions.

A final so what?

Many nursing leaders today, when asked, argue that the single most pressing issue facing practising nurses is their need to be able to articulate their activities and provide evidence of their effectiveness. Without this, the profession can have no assurance of a future. There is sometimes frustration at nurses' failure to unstop their ears to this warning of their demise. Like some of the hesitant middle managers involved in this study, I find the ground upon which to stand in order to question these arguments extremely narrow. One difficulty is that many in prominent and other leading positions are often already politically committed to preserving or advancing nursing, so that any truth claims are weighed up against the criteria of their place within this project. To suggest that a focus on visibility and the articulation of accountability may involve unforeseen consequences can be received as either an unhelpful comment or a nonstatement. Many nurses in leadership emphasise the need to speak in 'language that managers can understand' about the effect and hence the purpose of nursing. This may have the result that no one is speaking any other language. Those who could be challenging the less strident but still far-reaching effects of managerialism (by this I mean that 'macho-management' has been attacked far more than managerialism's rationality) are failing to present any alternative values.

I hope that this work may be of use to individuals like those involved in this research who were troubled by the changes affecting their work but found the language with which to articulate their feelings all but unavailable. They felt that it was impossible to criticise a managerial project which was so well defined and rational, and presented as an attempt to address notoriously difficult issues. Some nurses in 'middle-management' positions come first to mind. It is for these individuals and groups, who are becoming increasingly marginalised within nursing itself, that this account of the way that a particular discourse has been put into operation has been offered.

This book is a move in a continual agonistics, a challenge to the evangelists of modernity. It is a reminder that there are opposing discourses within this large organisation called the NHS (and in society at large) and that not all are convinced by the language of rationality.

The book is also a gesture of solidarity with those who suffer, subtly or overtly, under various regimes of control (perhaps this includes executives as much as community nurses), especially when that control wears a mask of rationality, consensus, development, of penetrating compassion, of acting-in-our-own-best-interests, warning us of our fate, robbing us of any basis of criticism and leaving only refusal.

I offer this work as a theoretical approach within which to mount offensives on totalising regimes, so that its arguments might be taken, developed, and used in other situations. This is a waging of war on totality.

References

Adorno, T. and Horkheimer, A. (1979) *Dialectic of Enlightenment*, London: Verso.

Adorno, T. and Horkheimer, A. (1996) 'The concept of Enlightenment; from *Dialectic of Enlightenment*', in *The Continental Philosophy Reader*, eds R. Kearney and M. Rainwater, London: Routledge.

Alexander, L., Sandridge, J. and Moore, L. (1993) 'Patient satisfaction: an outcome measure for maternity services', *Journal of Perinatal and Neonatal Nursing* 7(2): 28–29.

Allen, D. (1997) 'Nursing, knowledge and practice', *Journal of Health Services Research and Policy, Edinburgh* 2(3): 190–193.

Althusser, L. (1971) *For Marx*, London: Allen Lane.

Ashley, J. (1980) 'Misogny in medicine', *Advances in Nursing Science* 2(3): 3–22.

Atkinson, P. (1990) *The Ethnographic Imagination. Textual Constructions of Reality*, London: Routledge.

Atkinson, P. (1995) *Medical Talk and Medical Work: The Liturgy of the Clinic*, London: Sage.

Audit Commission (1991) *The Virtue of Patients: Making the Best Use of Nursing Resources*, London: HMSO.

Audit Commission (1992) *Community Care. Managing the Cascade of Change*, London: HMSO.

Audit Commission (1996a) *Fundholding Facts: A Digest of Information About Practices Within the Scheme During the First Five Years*, London: HMSO.

Audit Commission (1996b) *What the Doctor Ordered*, London: HMSO.

Austin, J. (1962) *How To Do Things With Words*, London: Oxford University Press.

Ball, J. (1991) 'Valuing nursing: a literature review', *Senior Nurse* 11(4): 23.

Baly, M. (1986) 'The Nightingale reform and hospital architecture', *History of Nursing Group at the Royal College of Nursing Bulletin* 11: 1–7.

Barthes, R. (1972) *Mythologies*, Frogmore: Granada.

Barthes, R. (1977) *Image, Music, Text*, New York: Hill & Wang.

Barthes, R. (1985) *The Fashion System*, London: Cape.

Barthes, R. (1996) 'Inaugural lecture at the College de France', in *The Continental Philosophy Reader*, eds R. Kearney and M. Rainwater, London: Routledge. 364–377.

Bartlett, W. and Le Grand, J. (1994) 'The performance of Trusts', in *Evaluating the NHS Reforms*, ed. R. Robinson and J. Le Grand, London: King's Fund Institute. 54–73.

Bell, D. (1985), *The Social Sciences Since the Second World War*, London: Transaction Books.

Benhabib, S. (1990) 'Epistemologies of the postmodern', in *Feminism/Postmodernism*, ed. L. Nicholson, London: Routledge. 107–130.

Benner, P. (1984) *From Novice to Expert: Excellence and Power in Clinical Nursing Practice*, Menlow Park, CA: Addison-Wesley.

Benner, P. and Wrubel, J. (1989) *The Primacy of Caring: Stress and Coping in Health and Illness*, Menlow Park CA: Addison-Wesley.

Bennet, G. (1987) *The Wound and the Doctor*, London: Secker & Warburg.

Bloom, H. (ed.) (1987) *The Bible. Edited and with an Introduction by Harold Bloom*, New York: Chelsea House.

Bloomfield, B., Coombs, R., Cooper, D. and Rea, D. (1992) 'Machines and manoeuvres: responsibility accounting and the construction of hospital information', *Accounting, Management and Information Technologies* 2(4): 199.

Brindle, D. (1995) 'Minister says £120m surplus is evidence of fundholding success', *Guardian*, 17 March.

Brown, P. and Sparks, R. (1989) 'Introduction', in *Beyond Thatcherism: Social Policy, Politics and Society*, eds P. Brown and R. Sparks, Milton Keynes: Open University Press.

Buchan, J. and Ball, J. (1991) *Caring Costs*, Sussex: Institute of Manpower Studies, University of Sussex.

Butler, J. (1992) *Patients, Policies and Politics: Before and After 'Working for Patients'*, Milton Keynes: Open University Press.

Callon, M., Law, J. and Rip, A. (eds) (1986) *Mapping the Dynamics of Science and Technology*, Basingstoke: Macmillan.

Canguilhem, G. (1969) *La Connaissance de la Vie*, Paris: Vrin.

Capra, F. (1983) *The Turning Point*, New York: Bantam Books.

Car-Hill, R., Dixon, P. and Griffiths, M. (1992) *Skill Mix and the Effectiveness of Nursing Care*, York: Centre for Health Economics, University of York.

Chandler, J. (1991) 'Reforming nurse education 1. The reorganisation of nursing knowledge', *Nurse Education Today* 11(2): 83–88.

Chinn, P. and Wheeler, C. (1985) 'Feminism and nursing: can nursing afford to remain aloof from the women's movement?', *Nursing Outlook* 33(2): 76.

Chodorow, N. (1978) *The Reproduction of Mothering: Psychoanalysis and the Sociology of Gender*, Berkeley: University of California Press.

Cixous, H. (1993) 'We who are free, are we free?', *Critical Inquiry* 19(2): 201–218.

Clay, T. (1987) *Nurses: Power and Politics*, London: Heinemann.

Cohen, L. (1993) *Beautiful Losers*, London: Black Spring Press.

Committee on Nursing (1972) *Report of the Committee on Nursing (Chairman: Asa Briggs)*, London: HMSO. Cmnd 5115.

Culler, J. (1983) *On Deconstruction: Theory and Criticism after Structuralism*, London: Routledge.

Davies, C. (1995) *Gender and the Professional Predicament in Nursing*, Buckingham: Open University Press.

De Beauvoir, S. (1953) *The Second Sex*, London: Cape.

de Man, P. (1979) *Allegories of Reading: Figurative language in Rousseau, Nietzsche, Rilke, and Proust*, New Haven, CT: Yale University Press.

De Saussure, F. (1974) *Course in General Linguistics*, London: Fontana.

De Saussure, F. (1996) 'Selections from the course in general linguistics', in *The Continental Philosophy Reader*, eds R. Kearney and M. Rainwater, London: Routledge. 291–304.

Deleuze, G. and Guattari, F. (1984) *Anti-Oedipus: Capitalism and Schizophrenia*, London: Athlone Press.

Denzin, N. and Lincoln, Y. (eds) (1994) *Handbook of Qualitative Research*, Newbury Park, CA: Sage.

Department of Health (1989a), *Caring for People*, London: HMSO.

Department of Health (1989b) *A Strategy for Nursing. A Report of the Steering Committee*, London: Department of Health Nursing Division.

Department of Health (1989c) *Working for Patients: Working Paper 10*, London: HMSO. Cmd. 555.

Department of Health (1991) *The Patient's Charter*, London: HMSO.

Department of Health (1996a) *The National Health Service: A Service with Ambitions*, London: Department of Health.

Department of Health (1996b) *Primary Care: The Future*, London: Department of Health.

Department of Health (1997) *The New NHS; Modern Dependable*, London: Department of Health. Cmd. 3807.

Department of Health and National Health Service Management Executive (1993) *A Vision for the Future. The Nursing, Midwifery and Health Visiting Contribution to Health and Health Care*, London: Department of Health.

Derrida, J. (1976) *Of Grammatology*, Baltimore: Johns Hopkins University Press.

Derrida, J. (1978) 'Speculating-On Freud', *Oxford Literary Review* 3: 78–97.

Derrida, J. (1982a) 'Signature event context', in *Margins of Philosophy*, Hemel Hempstead: Harvester Wheatsheaf. 307–330.

Derrida, J. (1982b) 'White mythology: metaphor in the text of philosophy', in *Margins of Philosophy*, Hemel Hempstead: Harvester Wheatsheaf. 207–272.

Derrida, J. (1992) 'Interview with Derrida', in *Logomachia*, ed. R. Rand, Lincoln: University of Nebraska Press. 195–218.

Drife, J. and Johnston, I. (1995) 'Management for doctors handling the conflicting cultures in the NHS', *British Medical Journal* 310(6986): 1054–1056.

Eagleton, T. (1983) *Literary Theory: An Introduction*, Oxford: Blackwell.

Ebert, T. (1988) 'The romance of patriarchy: ideology, subjectivity and postmodern feminist cultural theory', *Cultural Critique* 10: 19–57.

Edwards, J (1994). 'How to sell your services in the NHS', *Primary Health* 4(1): 6–8.

Enthoven, A. C. (1985). *Reflections on the Management of the National Health Service: An American Looks at Incentives to Efficiency in Health Services Management in the UK*, London: Nuffield Provincial Hospital Trust.

Fawcett, J. (1983) 'Contemporary nursing research: its relevance to nursing practice', in *The Nursing Profession: A Time to Speak*, ed. N. Chaska, New York: McGraw-Hill.

Fawcett, J. (1984) *Analysis and Evaluation of Conceptual Models of Nursing*, Philadelphia: F. A. Davis.

Ferlie, E. (1997) 'Large-scale organizational and managerial change in health care: a review of the literature', *Journal of Health Service Research and Policy, Edinburgh* 2(3): 180–189.

Foucault, M. (1965) *Madness and Civilisation. A History of Insanity in the Age of Reason.* New York, Pantheon.

Foucault, M. (1970) 'Las Meninas', in *The Order of Things: An Archaeology of the Human Sciences*, London: Routledge. 3–16.

Foucault, M. (1972) *The Archaeology of Knowledge*, London: Routledge.

Foucault, M. (1977) *Discipline and Punish*, Harmondsworth: Penguin.

Foucault, M. (1979) 'On governmentality', *Ideology and Consciousness* 6: 5–22.

Foucault, M. (1980a) 'The eye of power', in *Power/Knowledge. Selected Interviews and Other Writings 1972–1977*, ed. C. Gordon, Hemel Hempstead: Harvester Wheatsheaf. 146–165.

Foucault, M. (1980b) 'Two lectures', in *Power/Knowledge. Selected Interviews and Other Writings 1972–1977*, ed. C. Gordon, Hemel Hempstead: Harvester Wheatsheaf. 78–108.

Foucault, M. (1983) *This is Not a Pipe*, Berkeley: University of California Press.

Foucault, M. (1984a) *The History of Sexuality: Volume 1. An Introduction*, Harmondsworth: Penguin.

Foucault, M. (1984b) 'What is Enlightenment?', in *The Foucault Reader*, ed. P. Rabinow. Harmondsworth: Penguin. 32–50.

Foucault, M. (1986). *The History of Sexuality: Volume 3. The care of the self*. New York, Pantheon.

Foucault, M. (1989) *The Order of Things: An Archaeology of the Human Sciences*, London: Routledge.

Fox, N. (1993) *Postmodernism, Sociology and Health*, Buckingham: Open University Press.

Fraser, N. and Nicholson, L. (1990) 'Social criticism without philosophy', in *Feminism/Postmodernism*, ed. L. Nicholson, New York: Routledge. 19–38.

Freud, S. (1953) *A Difficulty in the Path of Psychoanalysis. Standard Edition*, London: Hogarth Press.

Fuller, S. (1978) 'Holistic man and the science and practice of nursing', *Nursing Outlook* 26: 700–704.

Gahmberg, H. (1990) 'Metaphor management: on the semiotics of strategic leadership', in *Organizational Symbolism*, ed. B. Turner, Berlin: Walter de Gruyter. 151–158.

Garfinkel, H. (1967) *Studies in Ethnomethodology*, Englewood Cliffs: Prentice-Hall.

Giddens, A. (1992) *The Transformation of Intimacy*, Cambridge: Polity Press.

Gilligan, C. (1982) *In a Different Voice: Psychological Theory and Women's Development*, London: Harvard University Press.

Goodman, C. (1989) 'Nursing research: growth and development', in *Current Issues in Nursing*, eds M. Jolley and P. Allan, London: Chapman & Hall. 95–114.

Gray, A. and Jenkins, B. (1993) 'Markets, management and the public service: the changing of a culture', in *Markets and Managers: New Issues in the Delivery of Welfare*, eds P. Taylor-Gooby and R. Lawson, Buckingham: Open University Press. 9–23.

Greenwood, J. (1984) 'Nursing research: a position paper', *Journal of Advanced Nursing* 9(1): 77–82.

Griffiths, R. (1983) *Report of the NHS Management Inquiry*, London: Department of Health and Social Security.

Habermas, J. (1984) *Theory of Communicative Action*, London: Heinemann Education.

Hagell, E. (1989) 'Nursing knowledge: women's knowledge. A sociological perspective', *Journal of Advanced Nursing* 14(3): 226–233.

Ham, C. (1991) *The New National Health Service: Organisation and Management*, Oxford: Radcliffe Medical Press.

Hammersley, M. (1995) *The Politics of Social Research*, London: Sage.

Hancock, C. (1998) 'Making decisions for patients', *Nursing Standard* 12(31): 20.

Harding, S. (1990) 'Feminism, science and the anti-Enlightenment critiques', in *Feminism/Postmodernism*, ed. L. Nicholson, New York: London: Routledge. 83–106.

Harrison, S., Hunter, D., Marnoch, G. and Pollitt, C. (1989) 'General management and medical autonomy in the National Health Service', *Health Services Management Research* 2(1): 38–46.

Harrison, S., Hunter, D., Marnock, G. and Pollitt, C. (1992) *Just Managing: Power and Culture in the NHS*, London: Macmillan.

Harrison, S., Hunter, D. and Pollitt, C. (1990) *The Dynamics of British Health Policy*, London: Unwin Hyman.

Harrison, S. and Pollitt, C. (1994) *Controlling Health Professionals: The Future of Work and Organisation in the NHS*, Buckingham: Open University Press.

Hart, C. (1994) *Behind the Mask: Nurses, Their Unions and Nursing Policy*, London: Balliere Tindall.

Hartsock, N. (1990) 'Foucault on power: a theory for women?', in *Feminism/ Postmodernism*, ed. L. Nicholson, New York: Routledge. 157–175.

Hayek, F. (1967) 'The moral element in free enterprise', in *Studies in Philosophy, Politics and Economics*, London: Routledge & Kegan Paul.

Health News (1994) '"More home visits" say mums', *Health Visitor* 67(9): 284.

Heckman, S. (1986) *Hermeneutics and the Sociology of Knowledge*, Cambridge: Polity Press.

Hegel, G. (1977) *Phenomenology of Spirit*, Oxford: Clarendon Press. First published 1807.

Heidegger, M. (1962) *Being and Time*, New York: Harper & Row.

Holliday, I. (1992) *The NHS Transformed*, Manchester: Baseline Books.

Holmes, C. (1990) 'Alternatives to natural science foundations for nursing', *International Journal of Nursing Studies* 27(3): 187–198.

Horkheimer, M. (1972) 'Traditional and critical theory', in *Critical Theory Selected Essays*, New York: Seabury Press.

HSJ News (1994) 'In Brief', *Health Service Journal* 104(7 April): 4.

HSJ News Focus (1996) 'News Focus', *Health Service Journal* 106(5493): 11.

Hughes, D. and Dingwall, R. (1990) 'What's in a name?', *Health Service Journal* 100: 1770–1771.

Johns, C. (1995) 'The value of reflective practice for nursing', *Journal of Clinical Nursing* 4(1): 23–30.

Johnson, D (1974) 'Development of theory: a requisite for nursing as a primary health profession', *Nursing Research* 23(5): 372–377.

Johnson, T. (1995) 'Governmentality and the institutionalization of expertise', in *Health Professions and the State in Europe*, eds T. Johnson, G. Larkin and M. Saks, London: Routledge.

Jolley, M. and Allan, P. (eds) (1991) *Current Issues in Nursing*, London: Chapman & Hall.

Jones, A. and Hendry, C. (1992) *The Learning Organisation: A Review of Literature and Practice*, London: HRD Partnership.

Jordanova, L. (1989) *Sexual Visions. Images of Gender in Science and Medicine between the Eighteenth and Twentieth Centuries*, Hemel Hempstead: Harvester Wheatsheaf.

Kant, I. (1784) cited in Foucault, M. (1984). 'What is Enlightenment?' *The Foucault Reader*, ed. P. Rainbow. Harmondsworth: Penguin. 32–50.

Kanigel, R. (1997) *The One Best Way: Frederick Winslow Taylor and the Enigma of Efficiency*, London: Little, Brown and Company.

Kelly, M. and Glover, I. (1996) 'In search of health and efficiency: the NHS 1948–94', in *Beyond Reason? National Health Service and the Limits of Management*. (Stirling Management Series), eds J. Leopold, M. Glover and M. Hughes, Aldershot: Avebury.

Kincheloe, J. and McLaren, P. (1994) 'Rethinking critical theory and qualitative research', in *Handbook of Qualitative Research*, eds N. Denzin and Y. Lincoln, Newbury Park, CA: Sage. 138–157.

Kitson, A. (ed.) (1993) *Nursing: Art and Science*, London: Chapman & Hall.

Klein, R. (1989) *The Politics of the National Health Service*, London: Longman.

Klevit, H., Bates, A., Castanares, T., Kirk, P., Sipes-Metzler, P. and Wopat, R. (1991) 'Prioritization of health care services. A progress report by the Oregon Health Services Commission', *Archives of International Medicine* 151(May 1991): 912–916.

Kuhn, T. (1970) *The Structure of Scientific Revolutions*, Chicago: Chicago University Press.

Lacan, J. (1980) *Ecrits/ Jacques Lacan: A Selection Translated from the French by Alan Sheridan*, London: Tavistock.

Lather, P. (1986) 'Research as praxis', *Harvard Educational Review* 56(3): 257–277.

Lather, P. (1991) *Getting Smart. Feminist Research and Pedagogy With/in the Postmodern*, London: Routledge.

Latimer, J. (1995) 'The nursing process re-examined: diffusion or translation?', *Journal of Advanced Nursing* 22: 213–220.

Latimer, J. (1997a) 'Giving patients a future: the constituting of classes in an acute medical unit', *Sociology of Health and Illness* 19: 160–185.

Latimer, J. (1997b) 'Organizing context: nurses' assessments of older people in an acute medical unit', *Nursing Inquiry* 5(12): 43–57.

Latour, B. (1987) *Science in Action*, Milton Keynes: Open University Press.

Latour, B. (1993) *We Have Never Been Modern*, Hemel Hempstead: Harvester Wheatsheaf.

Lawler, J. (1991) *Behind the Screens: Nursing, Somology and the Problem of the Body*, London: Churchill Livingstone.

Lawson, N. (1996) 'Is it the end, nurses?', *The Times*, 26 December.

Leininger, M. (1978) *Transcultural Nursing. Concepts, Theories and Practices*, New York: Wiley.

Leininger, M. (ed.) (1985) *Qualitative Research Methods in Nursing*, Orlando: Grune and Stratton.

Leininger, M. (1990) 'Historic and epistemologic dimensions of care and caring with future directions', in *Knowledge about Care and Caring*, eds J. S. Stevenson and T. Tripp-Reimer, Kansas City, MO: American Academy of Nursing. 19–31.

Levinas, E. (1996) 'Ethics as first philosophy', in *The Continental Philosophy Reader*, eds R. Kearney and M. Rainwater, London: Routledge. 124–135.

Lightfoot, J., Baldwin, S. and Wright, K. (1992) *Nursing by Numbers? Setting Staffing Levels for District Nursing and Health Visiting Services*, York: SPRU, University of York.

Lowe, R. (1990) 'Defending your territory', *Nursing Standard* 4(43): 50.

Lukes, S. (1994) *Power: A Radical View*, London: Macmillan.

Lupton, D. (1995) 'D & S forum: postmodernism and critical discourse analysis', *Discourse and Society* 6(2): 301–304.

Lyotard, J.-F. (1979) *The Postmodern Condition: A Report on Knowledge*, Manchester: Manchester University Press.

McBride, G. (1992). 'Bush vetoes health care rationing in Oregon' *British Medical Journal* 305(22 August 1992): 437.

McClarey, M. and Duff, L. (1997) 'Clinical effectiveness and evidence-based practice', *Nursing Standard* 11(52): 33–35.

MacIntyre, A. (1985) *After Virtue. A Study in Moral Theory*, London: Duckworth.

Macleod Clark, J. and Hockey, L. (1981) *Research for Nursing: A Guide for the Enquiring Nurse*. New York: John Wiley.

Marx, K. and Engels, F. (1969) *The German Ideology*. New York: International Publishers.

Mason, C. (1991) 'Project 2000: A critical review', *Nursing Practice* 4(3): 3.

Masterson, A. (1996) 'Primary nursing: New Right discourse in action?', paper given at Nursing, Women's History and the Politics of Welfare Conference, University of Nottingham.

Maynard, A. (1993) 'The economics of rationing health care', in *Rationing of Health Care in Medicine*, ed. M. Tunbridge. London: Royal College of Physicians. Ch. 1.

Maynard, D. (1989) 'On the ethnography and analysis of discourse in institutional settings', *Perspectives on Social Problems* 1: 127–146.

Meleis, A. (1985) *Theoretical Nursing: Development and Progress*, Philadelphia: J B Lippincott.

Melia, K. (1981) 'Communication in nursing. 3. Student nurses' construction of nursing: a discussion of a qualitative method', *Nursing Times* 77(16): 697–699.

Menzies, I. (1960) *A Case Study in the Functioning of Social Systems as a Defence Against Anxiety*. London: Tavistock.

Mercer, G. (1979) *The Employment of Nurses. Nursing Labour Turnover in the NHS*, London: Croom Helm.

Miller, J. (1993) *The Passion of Michel Foucault*, London: HarperCollins.

Miller, J. H. (1976) 'Steven's rock and criticism as cure', *The Georgia Review* 30: 5–31, 330–348.

Ministry of Health (1966) *Report of the Committee on Senior Nursing Staff Structure* (The Salmon Report), London: HMSO.

Morse, J. and Field, P. (1996) *Nursing Research: The Application of Qualitative Approaches*, London: Chapman & Hall.

Naish, J (1994). 'Editorial', *Nurses in Management* 1(1): 3.

National Audit Office (1992) *Nursing Education. Implementation of Project 2000 in England. Report by the Comptroller and Auditor General*, London: HMSO.

Newchurch (1995) *Sharpening the Focus: The Roles and Perceptions of Nursing in NHS Trusts*. London: Newchurch.

NHSME (1992a) *The Nursing Skill Mix in the District Nursing Service*, London: HMSO.

NHSME (1992b) *One Year On: The Nurse Executive Director Post. Report on the Role and Function of the Nurse Executive Director Post in First Wave NHS Trusts*, London: Department of Health and the Central Office of Information.

NHSME (1993) *New World, New Opportunities. Nursing in Primary Health Care*, London: National Health Service Management Executive.

Nicholson, L. (ed.) (1990) *Feminism/Postmodernism*, London: Routledge.

Nicholson, L. (1992) 'On the postmodern barricades: feminism, politics, and theory', in *Postmodernism and Social Theory*, eds S. Seidman and D. Wagner, Oxford: Blackwell. 82–100.

Nietzsche, F. (1967) *The Will to Power*, New York: Random House.

Nietzsche, F. (1994) *On the Genealogy of Morality*, Cambridge: Cambridge University Press.

Nightingale, F. (1883) *Notes On Hospitals*, London: Longman Green.

Norris, C. (1990a) 'Settling accounts: Heidegger, de Man and the ends of philosophy', in *What's Wrong with Postmodernism: Critical Theory and the Ends of Philosophy*, Hemel Hempstead: Harvester Wheatsheaf. 222–283.

Norris, C. (1990b) *What's Wrong with Postmodernism: Critical Theory and the Ends of Philosophy*, Hemel Hempstead: Harvester Wheatsheaf.

Norris, C. (1991). *Deconstruction: Theory and Practice*, London: Routledge.

North, N. and Porter, E. (1991) 'All change ahead', *Nursing Times* 87(3): 57–59.

Nozick, R. (1974) *Anarchy, State and Utopia*, New York: Basic Books.

Nursing Standard News (1992a) 'Move to defuse practice nurses' fears over GPs', *Nursing Standard* 6(19): 6.

Nursing Standard News (1992b) 'News', *Nursing Standard* 6(49): 13.

Nursing Times News (1990) 'Hancock urges positive outlook on reforms: speech at Primary Health Care Conference, November 1990', *Nursing Times* 86(45): 6.

Nutting, M. and Dock, L. (1907) *A History of Nursing: The Evolution of Nursing Systems from the Earliest Times to the Foundation of the First English and American Training Schools*, London: G P Putnam's sons.

Owens, P. and Glennerster (1990) *Nursing in Conflict*, Basingstoke: Macmillan.

Parker, I. (1992) *Discourse Dynamics: Critical Analysis for Social and Individual Psychology*, London: Routledge.

Parker, J. (1993) 'Toward a nursing ethic for sustainable planetary health', paper given at Health and Ecology – A Nursing Perspective. The First National Nursing the Environment Conference, Melbourne, Australia.

Parsons, C. (1995) 'The impact of postmodernism on research methodology: implications for nursing', *Nursing Inquiry* 2: 22–28.

Parsons, T. and Fox, R. (1952) 'Illness, therapy and the modern American family', *Journal of Social Issues* 8: 31–44.

Peters, T. and Waterman, R. (1982) *In Search of Excellence*, New York: Harper & Row.

Peterson, L. H. (1992) 'Deconstruction and Wuthering Heights' in *Wuthering Heights – Emily Bronte. Case Studies in Contemporary Criticism*, ed. L. H. Peterson, London: Macmillan.

Pollitt, C. (1991) *The politics of quality: managers, professionals and consumers in the public services. Revised version of a public lecture*. Royal Holloway and Bedford New College, Egham, Surrey: Royal Holloway and Bedford New College, Centre for Political Studies.

Pollitt, C. (1993) *Managerialism and the Public Services*, Oxford: Blackwell.

Potter, J. and Wetherell, M. (1987) *Discourse and Social Psychology: Beyond Attitudes and Behaviour*, London: Sage.

Prentice, S. (1991) 'What will we find at the market?', *Health Visitor* 65(1): 9–11.

Pringle, R. (1988) *Secretaries Talk. Sexuality, Power and Work*, London: Unwin.

Rabinow, P. (ed.) (1984) *The Foucault Reader*, Harmondsworth: Penguin.

Rafferty, A. M. (1992) 'Historical perspectives', in *Knowledge for Nursing Practice*, eds K. Robinson and B. Vaughan, Oxford: Butterworth-Heinemann.

Rafferty, A. M. (1993a) 'Decorous didactics: early explorations in the art and science of caring c. 1860–90', in *Nursing: Art and Science*, ed. A. Kitson, London: Chapman & Hall. 48–84.

Rafferty, A. M. (1993b) *Leading Questions: A Discussion Paper on the Issues of Nurse Leadership*, London: Kings Fund Centre.

Rathbone, W. (1892) 'Evidence to the select committee of the House of Lords on Metropolitan hospitals', *Parliamentary Papers* XIII.I: xci.

Renkema, J. (1993) *Discourse Studies: An Introductory Textbook*, Amsterdam: John Benjamins B.V.

Reverby, S. (1987) 'A caring dilemma: womanhood and nursing in historical perspective', *Nursing Research* 36(1): 5–11.

Richards, T. and Richards, L. (1994) Non-numerical Unstructured Data Indexing, Searching and Theorising (NUD•IST), Melbourne: Qualitative Solutions and Research Pty. Ltd.

Ricoeur, P. (1986) *The Rule of Metaphor. Multi-disciplinary Studies of the Creation of Meaning in Language*, London: Routledge.

Ricoeur, P. (1996) 'On interpretation', in *The Continental Philosophy Reader*, eds R. Kearney and M. Rainwater, London: Routledge. 136–155.

Rogers, M. (1980) 'Nursing: a science of unitary man', in *Conceptual Models for Nursing Practice*, eds J. P. Rheil and C. Roy, New York: Appleton-Century-Crofts.

Rorty, R. (1980) *Philosophy and the Mirror of Nature*, Princeton: Princeton University Press.

Rorty, R. (1989) *Contingency, Irony and Solidarity*, Cambridge: Cambridge University Press.

Rorty, R. (1991a) 'Cosmopolitanism without emancipation: a response to Jean-Francois Lyotard', in *Objectivity, Relativism, and Truth: Philosophical Papers Volume 1*, Cambridge: Cambridge University Press. 211–222.

Rorty, R. (1991b) 'Inquiry as recontextualisation: an anti-dualist account of inter-pretation', in *Objectivity, Relativism and Truth: Philosophical Papers*, Cambridge: Cambridge University Press. 93–110.

Rorty, R. (1991c) 'Science as solidarity', in *Objectivity, Relativism and Truth: Philosophical Papers Volume 1*, Cambridge, Cambridge University Press.

Rorty, R. (1991d) 'Solidarity or objectivity?', in *Objectivity, Relativism and Truth: Philosophical Papers Volume 1*, Cambridge: Cambridge University Press. 21–34.

Royal College of Nursing (1992) *The Value of Nursing*, London: Royal College of Nursing.

Royal College of Nursing (1994) *Nurses and NHS Productivity. The Facts*, London: Royal College of Nursing.

Royal College of Nursing (1995) *RCN Review Body Evidence*, London: Royal College of Nursing.

Russell, B. (1991) *History of Western Philosophy*, London: Routledge.

Sacks, H., Schegloff, E. and Jefferson, G. (1974) 'The simplest systematics for the organisation of turn-taking in conversation', *Language* 50: 697–735.

Said, E. (1978) *Orientalism*, New York: Pantheon.

Said, E. (1993) *Culture and Imperialism. The World, the Text and the Critic*, London, Chatto & Windus.

Salvage, J. (1985) *The Politics of Nursing*, London: Heinemann.

Salvage, J. (1988) 'Professionalisation – or struggle for survival? A consideration of current proposals for the reform of nursing in the United Kingdom', *Journal of Advanced Nursing* 13(4): 515–519.

Schön, D. (1983) *The Reflective Practitioner: How Professionals Think in Action*, London: Temple Smith.

Seedhouse, D. (1993) *Ethics: The Heart of Health Care*, London: John Wiley.

Seedhouse, D. (1997) 'Is a socialist health service possible?', *Health Care Analysis* 5(3): 183.

Seibold, C., Richards, L. and Simon, D. (1994) 'Feminist method and qualitative research about midlife', *Journal of Advanced Nursing* 19: 394–402.

Seidel, J. (1988) The Ethnograph V. 3.0, Corvallis: Qualis Research Associates.

Seidman, S. and Wagner, D., (eds) (1992) *Postmodernism and Social Theory*, Oxford: Blackwell.

Shaw, B. (1994) 'The year in brief: April 1993–December 1993', in *The Health Services Year Book 1994*, ed. L. Robertson, London: The Institute of Health Services Management.

Silverman, D. (1997) *Discourses of Counselling: HIV Counselling as Social Interaction*, London: Sage.

Smith, D. (1974) 'Women's perspective as a radical critique of sociology', *Sociological Inquiry* 44: 7–13.

Spender, D. (1980) *Man made language*, London: Routledge & Kegan Paul.

Spurgeon, P. and Barwell, F. (1991) *Implementing Change in the NHS. A Guide for General Managers*, London: Chapman & Hall.

Stewart, R. (1996) 'Divided loyalties', *Health Service Journal* 106(5495): 30–31.

Strong, P. (1983) 'The rivals', in *The Sociology of the Professions: Lawyers, Doctors and Others*, eds R. Dingwall and P. Lewis, London: Macmillan.

Strong, P. and Robinson, J. (1990) *The NHS – Under New Management*, Milton Keynes: Open University Press.

Stumpf, S. (1993) *Socrates to Sartre. A History of Philosophy*, New York: McGraw-Hill.

Swales, J. and Rogers, P. (1995) 'Discourse and the projection of corporate culture: the mission statement', *Discourse and Society* 6(2): 223–242.

Taylor, F. W. (1911) *The Principles of Scientific Management*, New York: Harper & Brothers.

Taylor-Gooby, P. (1994) 'Postmodernism and social policy: a great leap backwards?', *Journal of Social Policy* 23(3): 385–404.

Thompson, J. (1984) *Studies in the Theory of Ideology*, Cambridge: Polity Press.

Traynor, M. (1993) 'The morale of the community nursing workforce: a study of three NHS Trusts. Year 2', The Daphne Heald Research Unit, Royal College of Nursing.

Traynor, M. (1995) 'The morale of the community nursing workforce: a study of three NHS Trusts. The managers' account', The Daphne Heald Research Unit, Royal College of Nursing.

Traynor, M. and Wade, B. (1992) 'The morale of the community nursing workforce: a study of four NHS Trusts. Year 1', Daphne Heald Research Unit, Royal College of Nursing.

Traynor, M. and Wade, B. (1994) The morale of the community nursing workforce: a study of three NHS Trusts. Year 3', Daphne Heald Research Unit, Royal College of Nursing.

Turner, B. (ed.) (1990), *Organisational Symbolism*, Berlin: Walter de Gruyter.

Turner, T. (1994) 'Bodies and anti-bodies: flesh and fetish in contemporary social theory', *Embodiment and Experience. The Existential Ground of Culture and Self*, ed. T. Csordas, Cambridge: Cambridge University Press. 27–47.

UKCC (1986) Project 2000: A New Preparation for Practice, UKCC.

Van de Ven, A. (1980) 'Problem solving, planning and innovation, part 1: test of programme planning method; part 2: speculations for theory and practice', *Human Relations Journal* 33 (November–December): 10–11.

Wade, B. (1991) Research proposal: the changing face of community care and its impact on older people and the nursing workforce, draft document for discussion, Daphne Heald Research Unit, Royal College of Nursing.

Wainwright, D. (1996) 'The best of both worlds', *Health Service Journal* 106(5487): 30–31.

Walby, S. and Greenwell, J. (1994) *Medicine and Nursing. Professions in a Changing Health Service*, London: Sage.

Walsh, B. and Middleton, J. (1984) *The Transforming Vision; Shaping a Christian World View*, Downers Grove, IL: Inter Varsity Press.

Watson, J. (1981) 'Nursing's Scientific Quest', *Nursing Outlook* 29: 413–416.

Watson, J. (1985) *Nursing: Human Science and Human Care*, Norwalk: Appleton-Century-Crofts.

Webb, C. (1993) 'Feminist research: definitions, methodology, methods and evaluation', *Journal of Advanced Nursing* 18: 416–423.

Winner, L. (1977) *Autonomous Technology*, Boston: MIT Press.

Wistow, G. (1992) 'The National Health Service', in *Implementing Thatcherite Policies: An Audit of an Era*, eds D. Marsh and R. Rhodes, Milton Keynes: Open University Press. 100–116.

Zlotnick, C. and Gould, P. (1993) 'Prenatal quality of life outcomes for a public health quality assurance system', *Journal of Nursing Care Quality* 7(3): 35–45.

Index